The Path to
Athletic Power

The M... **n**

for C ... **e**

Boyd Epley, CSCS, MSCC

Associate Athletic Director
University of Nebraska

D1342547

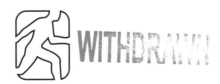
WITHDRAWN

Human Kinetics

Library of Congress Cataloging-in-Publication Data

Epley, Boyd.
  The path to athletic power : the model conditioning program for championship performance / Boyd Epley.
    p. cm.
  Includes index.
    ISBN 0-7360-4701-8 (soft cover)
    1. Physical education and training.   2. Physical fitness.   3. Epley, Boyd.   I. Title.
    GV711.5.E656   2004
    613.7'11--dc22

                                                                    2003024664
  ISBN: 0-7360-4701-8

The Web addresses cited in this text were current as of March 03, 2004, unless otherwise noted.

Developmental Editor: Laura Hambly; **Assistant Editor:** Carla Zych; **Copyeditor:** John Wentworth; **Proofreader:** Coree Clark; **Indexer:** Sharon Duffy; **Permission Manager:** Toni Harte; **Graphic Designer:** Nancy Rasmus; **Graphic Artists:** Sandra Meier and Tara Welsch; **Photo Managers:** Dan Wendt and Kelly Huff; **Cover Designer:** Keith Blomberg; **Photographer:** Front cover photos and photos on pages vi, 25, 28, 33, 50, 86, 171, 176, and 259 are used by permission of the Nebraska Athletic Department. All Nebraska Athletic Department logos and wordmarks included in the photos are property of the University of Nebraska Board of Regents. All other photos by Kelly Huff, unless otherwise noted; **Art Manager:** Kareema McLendon; **Illustrators:** Kareema McLendon (diagrams) and Mic Greenberg (medical art); **Printer:** United Graphics

We thank the University of Nebraska in Lincoln, Nebraska, for assistance in providing the location for the photo shoot for this book.

Human Kinetics books are available at special discounts for bulk purchase. Special editions or book excerpts can also be created to specification. For details, contact the Special Sales Manager at Human Kinetics.

Printed in the United States of America   10   9   8   7   6   5   4   3   2   1

Human Kinetics
Web site: www.HumanKinetics.com

United States: Human Kinetics
P.O. Box 5076
Champaign, IL 61825-5076
800-747-4457
e-mail: humank@hkusa.com

Canada: Human Kinetics
475 Devonshire Road Unit 100
Windsor, ON N8Y 2L5
800-465-7301 (in Canada only)
e-mail: orders@hkcanada.com

Europe: Human Kinetics
107 Bradford Road
Stanningley
Leeds LS28 6AT, United Kingdom
+44 (0) 113 255 5665
e-mail: hk@hkeurope.com

Australia: Human Kinetics
57A Price Avenue
Lower Mitcham, South Australia 5062
08 8277 1555
e-mail: liaw@hkaustralia.com

New Zealand: Human Kinetics
Division of Sports Distributors NZ Ltd.
P.O. Box 300 226 Albany
North Shore City
Auckland
0064 9 448 1207
e-mail: blairc@hknewz.com

For 34 years I had the privilege of working with exceptional young men and women who came to the University of Nebraska to participate in their chosen sport. My success as a strength coach was a reflection of their hard work. You can't always tell at the time if you're reaching them or having the influence that you'd like. Former Huskers football coach Tom Osborne always said it was the relationships with his athletes that were most rewarding for him, not the wins. You never really realize what an impact you might have on someone. Fortunately, I have been a strength coach long enough that many athletes have had the opportunity to come back and share their feelings with me. I understand what Coach Osborne was talking about. I dedicate this book to the Nebraska athletes and thank them for their belief in the Husker Power program and for choosing to be a part of the Husker Nation.

Contents

Foreword

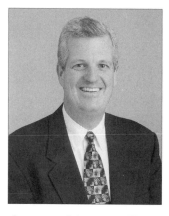

It was an unlikely setting, but that's often where we discover the profound. It was a night before another nationally televised Cornhusker football game, this one on the road in a state many miles away from Nebraska. I asked for a tour of the university's new facilities. Our tour guide was an anxious strength coach eager to show us his beautiful new weight room. His excitement was heightened by the fact that I had Boyd Epley with me.

As we walked into the complex, it occurred to me what Boyd Epley has accomplished over the past 34 years. Here, in a weight room hundreds of miles away from Lincoln, his influence was truly evident. We all know about the great program at Nebraska and how Husker Power has served so many great teams over the years. But this was more than that.

The new weight room we were in was filled completely with equipment designed by Boyd and his staff. In the middle stood this talented young strength coach for whom Boyd had turned a job into a profession. And the program, of course, was modeled after Nebraska's.

This book is the story of a career path to athletic power but, more important, it's a story of a lifetime of impact.

Steve Pederson
Nebraska Athletic Director

Preface

Husker Power, the University of Nebraska's strength and conditioning program, illustrates the growth of sports conditioning in America. Before 1970, weightlifting was not recommended for athletes in team sports. Many people believed that lifting weights would make athletes muscle bound and slower. At the time, Olympic weightlifting, powerlifting, and bodybuilding were the few choices athletes had if they wanted to lift weights. There were no strength coaches, as we know them today, to show athletes how to train with weights to improve performance. *The Path to Athletic Power* shows how innovations in strength and conditioning at Nebraska influenced sports conditioning across the country and helped create a profession of strength coaches.

One of the first All-Americans involved with Husker Power was Jerry Murtaugh. Jerry once asked me, "Boyd, why are you doing this? You get paid $2 an hour for two hours a day but you're here at least eight hours a day." I explained to Jerry that I had a vision that some day what I was doing would be a real profession that would really help athletes improve performance. Jerry didn't share the vision, at least not at the time. In fact, I think he thought I was crazy.

Twenty years later, Jerry returned to Nebraska, this time with his son Ryan, who was a football recruit. Jerry remembered the conversation he'd had with me about wasting my time as a strength coach and was quick to point out how impressed he was with how far Husker Power had come. Ironically, Jerry now is the driving force in raising money to help high schools in Omaha, Nebraska, hire strength coaches. His goal? To place a strength coach in every high school in Omaha.

Over the years, many skeptics like Jerry have seen the obvious benefits of sports conditioning and had to change their tune. They now realize there's no faster way to improve performance than through sports conditioning. In this book you'll find a comprehensive conditioning plan for athletes whose goal is to develop their potential to the fullest. You'll learn how to design a complete program, including in-season, off-season, and multisport programs. Chapters on testing, evaluation, and goal setting will get you going on making appropriate gains in strength, power, speed, and agility. Today's athletes are stronger and more explosive, with incredible speed and mobility—a far cry from the athletes of yesterday, who never heard of sports conditioning.

Not only have athletes changed—so has lifting equipment. Lifting facilities across the nation have developed and prospered beyond what anyone could have imagined in the 1950s or '60s. Nebraska is nationally known for its outstanding sports conditioning facilities. When people think of the right way to train athletes, they think of Nebraska first. *The Path to Athletic Power* gives you the information you need to design and implement a program like Nebraska's. You'll learn all the practical things—how to assess your program needs, determine your budget, select equipment, and organize your facility to best suit the needs of your athletes—but you'll also see for yourself how the success of a program depends almost entirely on the people behind it. With vision and enthusiasm, you can do nearly anything. You'll see the proof of this on every page of this book.

There are many other books on strength, conditioning, and nutrition, but I didn't want this book to be like those. I didn't want to write a typical reference book. I wanted a book that was fun to read, with true, behind-the-scenes stories that show you how to rise to success. Yes, you need to know all the sports conditioning concepts and the practical information on starting and running a program, but you also want to hear the human side of things. That's really what sets this book apart. In my time at Nebraska, I've met so many people who helped me at just the right time. In part, this book is a tribute to them. That's why you'll see them in these pages, the real people, some who went on to great fame and some who operate behind the scenes.

I hope you enjoy the read and benefit from it. By the end of the book, you'll know much better how to match a strength-training facility with a strength-conditioning program geared to improve performance.

The Advent of Formal Sports Conditioning

Remember Bob Beamon? The 1968 Olympic world-record long-jumper with the pencil-thin physique? Beamon stood 6 feet, 3 inches, and weighed all of 154 pounds. Or perhaps you recall the 1972 U.S. men's Olympic basketball team. A player on that team, Doug Collins, was 6 feet, 6 inches, and weighed 180 pounds. On the female side, think back to the slim frame of Peggy Fleming, Olympic gold medalist in figure skating. Or, moving to football, remember Rik Bonness, the two-time All-American center from Nebraska? Bonness weighed just 224 pounds—tiny by today's standards. Today, we have athletes such as Shaquille O'Neal, who plays basketball at 345 pounds, his shoulders as wide as a car. Strength and conditioning concerns are no longer limited to athletes in the traditional "power sports," such as football, basketball, and baseball. Today, golfers are lifting weights to gain muscle to hit the ball farther. A truck loaded with exercise equipment now regularly accompanies the PGA tour.

In 1900, the average All-American football lineman stood 6 feet, 1 inch, and weighed 195 pounds. By 1950, the average lineman was 6 feet, 2-1/2 inches, and 220 pounds. In 1984, average linemen were 6 feet, 4-1/2 inches, and 268 pounds. Clearly, athletes have become significantly larger over the last century. In 2002, a 14-year-old, 8th-grade elementary school basketball player in Fanwood, New Jersey, stood 6 feet, 9 inches, and weighed 286 pounds. Also in that year, the NFL introduced its first 400-pound offensive lineman—Aaron Gibson of the Dallas Cowboys, who stands 6 feet, 6 inches, and weighs 410 pounds. Soon, 400-pound athletes with great mobility and speed will be common in many sports, not just football.

Athletes are also getting stronger and more explosive. Doug Dumler, the starting center on Nebraska's 1970 NCAA national champion football team, was the only player on the team who could clean 300 pounds. Less than 30 years later, Nebraska's 1997 NCAA national championship team had a starting quarterback, Scott Frost, who could hang clean 300 pounds for *10* repetitions. Many female athletes today can clean over 300 pounds and leap 30-inch vertical jumps.

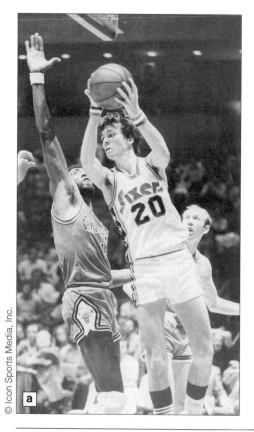
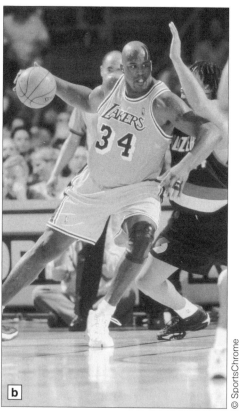

Compare the size and physique of *(a)* 1972 U.S. Olympic basketball player Doug Collins to *(b)* today's NBA player Shaquille O'Neal. Modern sports conditioning programs have produced stronger, more explosive athletes with outstanding speed and mobility.

Many sports coaches once believed that lifting weights made athletes muscle bound and inflexible. They believed lifting diminished coordination and might throw off the shot in basketball in some way. Today we know that there's no faster way to improve performance than through sports conditioning. Sports conditioning combines strength training with speed and agility drills. Strength training combines training methods from three sports: bodybuilding, weightlifting, and powerlifting. Athletes develop size through bodybuilding methods, gain power through explosive lifts, such as in Olympic weightlifting, and build strength through squats, as powerlifters do.

I introduced Nebraska athletes to the benefits of sports conditioning in 1969 and used my experience from competing in bodybuilding, Olympic weightlifting, and powerlifting to further develop the program in the early 1970s. Many colleges and high schools had already started lifting programs, but because I founded the National Strength and Conditioning Association (NSCA) in 1978, I had the good fortune of being recognized for helping to initiate sports conditioning for athletes in the United States. Today, many coaches are following suit and using methods from the disciplines of bodybuilding, weightlifting, and powerlifting to help their athletes reach their full potential.

Bodybuilding

My recommended program for athletes calls for three sets of 10 repetitions to build a base. Base training comes from the type of training used for bodybuilding. While competing in physique competitions in the early 1970s, I found that bodybuilders are generally concerned only with appearance, not performance. As a result, they usually aren't as strong as powerlifters or as explosive as Olympic weightlifters. However, the high repetitions bodybuilders perform as part of their training do have some carryover for athletes toward building muscle mass.

The first physique contest was held in New York's Madison Square Garden in 1903 (won by Albert Treloar) and was the only event of its type for more than 20 years. In 1939, the AAU (Amateur Athletic Union) held the first Mr. America contest, won by John Grimek. Training and competing at a time before steroids had been invented and vitamin supplementation was in its infancy, Grimek won the Mr. America competitions in 1939 and 1940 because of his tremendous natural physique.

In 1977, I was invited to help judge the Mr. America contest and participate in a parade featuring former Mr. America winners. Richard Countryman, the National Physique Chairman, asked if I was interested in replacing him as the national chairman, but I was so disappointed in what I saw in terms of drug use in the sport of bodybuilding that I declined any further involvement and turned my focus completely to sports conditioning.

Steroids ruined the sport of bodybuilding for me. Arnold Schwarzenegger, arguably the most popular bodybuilder, was a weightlifter in his younger days but switched to bodybuilding during a period plagued by steroids. Arnold dominated bodybuilding during this period before gaining fame as a movie star. After his bodybuilding career ended, he visited all 50 states at his expense on behalf of the President's Council on Physical Fitness, which had a big impact on the acceptance of strength training by the population in general. During his trip to Nebraska, Schwarzenegger gained many fans when he took time to say hello to players and coaches at football practice inside Memorial Stadium.

Few bodybuilders have a clean, good guy image, but one class act was Bill Pearl, who always set a good example for young bodybuilders. Steve Reeves was another of my favorites, winning the Mr. America and Mr. Universe at age 21 in 1947. The biggest or most muscular contestant doesn't always win the physique competition. Judges watch the posing routine and grade the presentation, and they also grade for symmetry and muscular development. It's very rare to see someone with the perfect symmetry Reeves had. He had 19-inch arms, a 19-inch neck, and 19-inch calves.

I'll explain this in more detail in chapter 4, but the objective of strength training for athletes is to build a base of muscular size. The process of building a base comes from bodybuilding. High-volume, low-intensity workouts like the ones bodybuilders do will increase muscle mass faster than low-volume, high-intensity workouts. Three sets of 10 repetitions for the first 4 weeks for a 12-week program is the recommended way to build muscle. The larger the muscle fibers become through strength training, the greater their capacity to apply force.

Olympic Weightlifting

Olympic-style weightlifting has great application for athletes in power sports. Great feats of strength are generally thought to be linked with outstanding athletic performances. But close examination of most sports shows that although strength is very important, power is even more important. Power combines speed and strength. For example, in the shot-put, the objective is to accelerate the shot as quickly as possible so that it's moving at maximum speed at release. The pitch in baseball works a similar way—many different body parts work together to produce a summation of forces so that during the final wrist and finger action the ball is traveling at maximum speed.

Speed of execution (explosiveness) is also very important in running and jumping. In running, the foot is in contact with the ground for about a 10th of a second. This means that in an extremely short amount of time the muscles of the leg must generate sufficient force to push the runner forward. In jumping, the foot contacts the ground during takeoff for about two to three 10ths of a second. Again, the pushoff is executed in an extremely short period of time. The key element is overcoming the resistance involved within the short time you have in order to execute the movement as quickly as possible. In building power—that is, speed *and* strength—weightlifting has huge consequences for athletes in sports such as football and basketball.

Weightlifting, because it's less convenient for most athletes, requires a strong commitment. If you go to a health club or recreation center, you'll probably see some bodybuilders and possibly some powerlifters, but it's unlikely you'll see any Olympic-style weightlifters because this type of lifting requires lifting platforms and bumper plates.

Weightlifting has been contested in all Olympics since 1896. Americans won two medals in 1904 but did not compete again until 1932. Bob Hoffman had a tremendous impact on the sport of weightlifting and has become known as the father of weightlifting in the United States. He was an active lifter himself and organized the famous York Barbell Club in 1932, where he recruited the best weightlifters to train with him. With Bob Hoffman as coach of the United States Olympic weightlifting team, the United States won three team titles. Some of the Olympic champions that contributed to America's success were Tommy Kono, Norbert Schemansky, John Davis, and Paul Anderson. But the weightlifting fortunes of the United States have taken a dramatic slide downward since 1956.

Mastering the demanding techniques of weightlifting takes years of training and access to the proper facilities. Louisiana State University was the first college program in which athletes used weightlifting to improve performance. Alvin Roy was an Olympic weightlifter who brought weightlifting to LSU football in the 1950s under head coach Paul Dietzel. A year after implementing Roy's weightlifting program, LSU went undefeated and won its first national championship in the fall of 1958. LSU's star running back Billy Cannon was drafted by the San Diego Chargers in 1959. Cannon told Sid Gillman, coach of the San Diego Chargers, about LSU's weightlifting program and how much it had helped their players. Coach Gillman invited Alvin Roy to apply his weightlifting program in San Diego, and the added explosiveness was like a secret weapon as the Chargers went on to win the American Football League championship.

Doug Dumler and Mike Beran, Nebraska's center and guard on the football team that won the 1970 national championship, were pioneers for Nebraska in competitive weightlifting. I did not encourage the entire team to train as weightlifters, but these two had an interest, so I assisted them in training for weightlifting competition. Dumler set four records as he won the 242-pound title and was named the outstanding lifter for the 1971 Nebraska Collegiate Olympic Championships. Beran, who finished behind Dumler in the 242-pound class in the 1971 Olympic meet, won both Olympic weightlifting and powerlifting titles in 1972.

One Thursday afternoon in November 1970, Jim Williams, my first assistant, said he was going to a lifting meet. I asked what type of meet, and he explained that a group of guys in Norfolk, headed by Dale Blattert, hosted Olympic-style lifting meets a few times a year. That sounded interesting to me because I really believed in the explosive action of the Olympic lifts, though I had never done snatches. Back then, the meet consisted of the press, the snatch, and the clean and jerk. I asked Mike Arthur, a freshman powerlifter, to watch my form as I tried the snatch lift. Mike and I basically learned how to do the snatch together that day. I managed 205 pounds with pretty shaky form the first day, but I decided to go along with Jim Williams and give it a try in an actual lifting meet two days later. I snatched 215 pounds in the meet and later learned the state snatch record for my weight class was 220 pounds.

Peary Rader and Mabel Rader were meet directors for many of the Olympic lifting meets and had a positive influence on me. They encouraged me to continue in Olympic lifting, which I did for three years. Eventually, I raised the state record to 270 pounds in the snatch. Peary owned *Iron Man* magazine and sold metric lifting equipment in Alliance, Nebraska. The University of Nebraska purchased its first metric set from Peary, which included black Eleiko rubber bumper plates. Before we had the bumper plates, we would drop the cast-iron weights on the cement floor. I remember our groundskeeper, Bill Sheppard, complaining about the noise from the athletes dropping the weights just above his office in the north fieldhouse. For several reasons, it's not a good idea to build a weight room on the second floor. The rubber bumper plates were a tremendous improvement from a noise standpoint and also helped motivate players to do hang cleans.

Our off-season program at Nebraska calls for two of our four days per week to focus on explosive movements from the Olympic lifting family of exercises. Most major university programs have what I call a "technician" on staff or a local expert on Olympic lifts. Rodger DeGarmo is our technician. Rodger was instrumental to the lifting set-up and warm-up area at the 1996 Olympics in Atlanta. Nebraska is fortunate to have him. Both our athletes and the other strength coaches benefit from his expertise. We require all student strength coaches to spend time with Rodger to learn the proper technique for explosive lifts. At some schools, the technician gets carried away, and the program becomes a training ground for weightlifters. When I hired Rodger, I asked him not to let that happen at Nebraska. Rodger is very capable of training weightlifters and has trained several national champions, but he believes in the Husker Power philosophy. There will always be a few athletes who want to pursue weightlifting and compete in meets, but what I'm after for our program is a blend of the best parts of bodybuilding, Olympic lifting, and powerlifting into a program that improves performance for athletes in their sport.

Powerlifting

Powerlifting doesn't require as much technique as Olympic weightlifting, and success can come very quickly. Consequently, powerlifting has become much more popular in the United States than Olympic weightlifting. All athletes, regardless of their sport, must develop strength first. We use powerlifting exercises to build strength.

The first national powerlifting meet was held in 1964 and the first world championship in 1971. The three powerlifts are the squat, bench press, and deadlift; the lifter with the highest total for the three wins in each weight class. The United States has dominated every world championship, with Larry Pacifico, John Cole, Lamar Gant, Mike Bridges, Dan Austin, Dr. Fred Hatfield, and Jan Todd (just to name a few) winning titles. Dan Austin was a master strength and conditioning coach at Oklahoma State University until 2002. He was voted the best powerlifter of all time for his weight class. His 730-pound squat and 730-pound deadlift are beyond imagination for someone weighing only 148 pounds.

In the sport of powerlifting, the object is to lift the maximum weight possible, regardless of how fast you can do it. Because maximum weights are lifted, movements are very slow—in fact, the movement is so slow sometimes that the lift resembles a static contraction (which has no movement). Because powerlifting involves only strength, with no dependency on speed, it would make more sense to call powerlifting "strength lifting." Power is the amount of work done over a set amount of time. For instance, if you lifted a 200-pound weight a distance of three feet in one second, your power would be equal to 600 watts. If you lifted the same amount of weight for the same distance but executed the lift in half a second, you would have exhibited 1,200 watts of power, and the movement would be more explosive.

The sport that displays the greatest amount of strength coupled with the greatest amount of speed is Olympic weightlifting. Weightlifting requires maximum strength and maximum speed. It involves quick, explosive-type movements executed in the shortest amount of time. It's well known that for maximum increases in strength, maximum weights in the 85 to 100 percent of maximum range must be used. But in training with maximum weights the way powerlifters do, the movements produce strength but are inevitably very slow and don't attempt to simulate athletes' performance in sport.

In training for speed, light weights (25 to 50 percent of maximum) and fast execution are used. However, with continuous use of only light weights and fast movements, strength decreases. In time, as strength diminishes, speed also decreases and movements become slower. In addition to experiencing this decrease in strength, you become more susceptible to injury. It's important to know that your objective is not strength alone but to develop explosiveness for success in sports. We call our strength coaches at Nebraska the "Performance Team" because we want to improve performance. The process involves developing strength, but our main objective is becoming more explosive.

With all the changes in strength training over the years, somewhere along the way, the bench press became the most popular exercise among athletic programs in the United States. I was on the bench press bandwagon for many years, promoting a bench press club and awarding T-shirts for levels of achievement. Our bench press club at Nebraska recognized athletes who could bench 300 pounds or more—but when, eventually, Lawrence Pete benched 500 pounds, we decided we were emphasizing this exercise too much. While the bench press remains popular, it doesn't have as much carryover value to athletics as ground-based exercises such as the squat and clean. When athletes are lying on their back with a board providing stabilization, it takes away from their development. To shift our emphasis, we eliminated the bench press from our record keeping and moved the records to the museum. In 2002, we started having football players do the NFL bench-press test, which calls for 225 pounds done for as many reps as possible in one set. It's a fun test and doesn't take long, and the players really like it. A former Nebraska lineman, Brendan Stai, holds the NFL record of 42 repetitions with 225 pounds.

I have been criticized for taking the bench press records down, but doing so accomplished exactly what I wanted it to—it put the emphasis on the squat and hang clean. Will Shields was a perfect example of a great athlete who had a very modest bench press. He was a three-year high school starter at Lawton, Oklahoma. He came to Nebraska as a 280-pound lineman with a bench press of 205 pounds, but he played great football. Relying on the strength of his legs and hips, Shields achieved enough success that he won the 1992 Outland trophy as the outstanding college lineman in the country. He did improve his bench press to 380 pounds as a senior, but compared to most linemen, he always had a modest bench press. It didn't matter. He helped the Huskers win national team rushing titles in three of his four seasons. Following his collegiate career, Shields was selected by the Kansas City Chiefs in the third round of the 1993 NFL draft and continues to enjoy a successful career, being selected to the Pro Bowl in each of the past seven seasons.

The fact is the bench press is overrated for most athletes. Sure, you need muscle mass development in the upper body, but a big bench press doesn't translate to athletic success.

The best bench presser I ever saw was Mike McDonald, who held the world bench press record in four different weight classes. At a regional powerlifting meet in Omaha, Nebraska, Mike McDonald was in the warm-up room, but he didn't look very athletic so no one was sure if he was entered in the meet or not. He was from Minnesota and had traveled to Omaha, where no one knew much about him. After my final lift of 390 pounds, everyone figured the meet was over, but this pudgy guy was still in the warm-up room. A meet official asked him if he was planning to lift, and he said yes. The official said, "Well, the bar is at 390 pounds, and all the other lifters are done." McDonald said he'd start at 400 pounds. He lowered the bar to his chest and drove it easily to full arms' length, much to the surprise of everyone, including me. He followed with an easy 425-pound bench press and finished at 450 pounds. No one in Nebraska had ever seen such strength, especially on someone who wasn't all that muscular. McDonald had been in the service, and this was his first competition in several years. He trained hard, and the next year he bench pressed 485 pounds at a body weight of 181 pounds for a new world record. He later added world records in the 198-, 220-, and 242-pound classes before he retired.

Strength Research

Until 1978 and the formation of the NSCA, most research that addressed physical conditioning was aerobic based. This was largely because of the influence of Dr. Kenneth Cooper and other exercise physiologists. The aerobic movement created a path for fitness, which was needed by the general public, but it had little to do with improving performance for athletes. Even today in health clubs you'll see rows and rows of treadmills for aerobic workouts and hundreds of machines that work single joints but no lifting platforms for athletes. Strength researchers such as Dr. Thomas DeLorme, Dr. Richard Berger, and Dr. Peter Karpovich presented much of the theory that sent athletes down the correct path to train with weights. Following World War II, DeLorme demonstrated the importance of "progressive resistance exercise" in increasing muscular strength and hypertrophy for the rehabilitation of military personnel.

It wasn't until current researchers Dr. John Garhammer, Dr. Michael Stone, Dr. Bill Kraemer, Dr. Steven Fleck, and others focused on strength research that athletes had a clearer path to athletic power. Dr. Kraemer says, "The common theme of most resistance training studies is that it must be progressive in order to produce substantial and continued increases in muscle strength and size." He says, "Husker Power leads the field in applying science to its program. The reason they're seeing the gains is they're taking advantage of the latest science" (Anderson 1996). Dr. Kraemer visited Nebraska in the early seventies when he was still the strength coach at Carroll College in Iowa. I put him through a circuit program we were calling the "survivor circuit." The program led to way too much lactic acid build-up because it didn't have enough rest built in. The athletes would do 10 repetitions in less than 20 seconds; then we'd give them 30 seconds to recover before they did their second set at the same station. They followed with a third set at each station before moving to the next station. Needless to say, this workout nearly killed Dr. Kraemer. We abandoned the program because it wasn't giving us the gains we wanted. Kraemer didn't forget about the program, however. He used it for the first NSCA-sponsored research project. As a result, he came up with the metabolic circuit presented in chapter 11. It's studies such as those by Dr. Kraemer and other researchers that furthered the development of sports conditioning and influenced strength coaches in creating the applications commonly used today. Presented in chapter 10 are the results of some training sessions for athletes who lifted but did not run and yet produced impressive gains in acceleration and speed. Zach Duval, a former Nebraska strength coach, proves in these sessions that you don't need to run to get faster.

Women in Sport

Women had a rocky journey getting to where they are in athletic competition as well as in their sports conditioning. Today, however, women train as hard and as often as men. It's hard to imagine that women were barred from participating in or even watching the original Olympic Games. In fact, doing so was an offense punishable by death. When Olympic competition started again in 1896, women were still not allowed to compete. About 85 years later, the NCAA began competitions for women, but women were not allowed to run a marathon in the Olympics until 1984. A myth that women were too frail for long distances led Olympic administrators to limit women's competitions to shorter distances. Also, for their protection, women were not allowed to pole-vault until 1996. Not surprisingly, young women quickly showed they were able to handle the strain. In 2002, a young woman in Nebraska vaulted over 13 feet to lead the nation's high school athletes. The women's world record in the pole-vault will soon top the 16-foot mark.

Today at most colleges and high schools, women have equal access to facilities to train and compete. Since 1975, their status has changed dramatically. *Sports Illustrated* reported that in 1999 women received

33 percent of NCAA budgets nationwide, 41 percent of the sports scholarships, and 30 percent of the recruiting dollars.

Of course, Nebraska was involved firsthand in this evolution of women in sport. In July 1975, Dr. Aleen Swofford was hired as Nebraska's first athletic director for women. Nebraska's 10 women's sports were governed by the Association of Intercollegiate Athletics for Women until 1982, when the NCAA began sanctioning women's sports. Until 1982, women were not allowed on the main level of the north fieldhouse, where the Nebraska athletic department weight room was located.

Things weren't much better around the nation in those days. Barbara Hedges, the athletic director at the University of Washington, can offer some perspective on the impact of Title IX. She was hired as associate athletic director at Southern California in 1973. At that time, "the entire women's program budget was $17,000. There were no full-time coaches and no scholarships, which was very typical of women's programs at that time" (2002).

At Nebraska, female students were not allowed in the basement of the coliseum, which meant that physical education weight-training classes were offered to male students only. I worked with Jake Geier of the physical education department to expand the student weight room in the coliseum from 2,500 square feet to 4,000 square feet and to allow access by female students in 1973.

In 1975, I started letting female athletes come in through the fire exit to use the football weight room in the north fieldhouse. Freshman Peggy Liddick was the first female athlete to be mentioned in my *Lifting* newsletter in March of 1976. She would become Nebraska's first female conference champion in 1978, winning the vault in gymnastics.

In 1989, Dr. Jim Griesen, Vice Chancellor for Student Affairs at Nebraska, increased the student weight room to 7,800 square feet and asked me to recommend the equipment layout design. The student weight room at Nebraska for a time was the second largest in the Big Eight conference, including all athletic weight rooms. We also created a small weight room in the coliseum to be used only by female athletes.

As women's training opportunities increased, their facilities did not keep pace. Terry Petitt, coach of Nebraska's national championship women's volleyball team in 1995, did not have access to shower facilities for his female athletes for the first 10 years he was volleyball coach (1977-1987), even though his team was the Big Eight champion each year. Gender equity was unheard of, despite the passage of Title IX in 1972. Looking to the future, I asked Nebraska to include a staff locker room for female strength coaches in 1981, though I did not have any female employees at the time. In 2002, I had four full-time female members on my Performance Team in addition to several female graduate and undergraduate student strength coaches.

Strength Programs for Men Versus Women

In sports involving speed, strength, and endurance, men generally excel over women. The lower strength levels of women when compared to men reflect a significant difference in body size and body composition. These are the primary reasons for the difference in athletic performance between men and women. At the age of 10, performance levels are about equal because body size and strength differences are minimal before puberty, but during puberty these differences begin to widen and become fully developed in adulthood.

On average, women are about 4 inches shorter and 30 pounds lighter than men. Women also tend to carry about 10 percent more body fat, which means that an average man's body composition consists of much more muscle in relation to fat than does an average woman's body. Because of greater muscle size and percentage of muscle, most men are stronger than most women. In fact, women have about two-thirds the strength of men. As a consequence, female athletes should not be expected to compete against men of the same body weight. Every once in a while you hear of a young female wrestler who is winning matches by beating males at her same weight class. This is really remarkable when you consider the physical advantages the boys have.

Women don't have the same capabilities men have in increasing muscular size. This is because the hormone testosterone, which contributes to muscular size, is present in quantities 10 times greater in the average male than in the average female. Although men have greater capabilities to increase in muscular size, women tend to lose more fat than men as a result of strength training.

While women are much weaker than men in the chest, shoulders, and arms, they compare more closely in leg and hip strength. The quality of muscle in both females and males in terms of the muscle's ability to exert force is the same. Coaches learned early on there was no need to devise special strength programs for females, because the same programs are equally effective for men and women. Of course there are certain areas to emphasize, depending on the circumstances, that sometimes involve gender. For instance, football players generally need to strengthen the neck, whereas female athletes need to strengthen the muscles associated with landing. Consequently, there are two areas of the strength program in which lifting for women is different than in the program for men. Neck exercises are included for football players but not for athletes in other sports, and landing drills are included for women's sports. The common belief is that because women have a wider pelvis, there's added stress on the femur, which puts torque on the knee joint. Landing drills are included in the exercise section of this book (chapter 11) to strengthen the muscles associated with landing.

Effects of Title IX

All schools know the importance of making sure the legal requirements of Title IX are fully adhered to. A consultant is hired every few years to evaluate Nebraska women's programs to ensure opportunities are equal to those of the men. The evaluation covers several areas that coaches need to pay attention to. The Title IX regulation requires that institutions provide equal athletic opportunities for both genders. For example, a school with a fieldhouse for football to use must have comparable space available for other sports as well. The government is looking for availability and quality in addition to equal treatment of men and women's sports.

- Equipment—This has to do with the quality of equipment for men's and women's teams and if it's appropriate for their needs. If the football team gets new strength equipment, and the used strength equipment goes to a weight room used for female sports, you have a gender equity problem. The process for ordering and maintaining equipment needs to be similar for all teams.

- Scheduling—The availability of the facility and the equipment stations needs to be equitable for all teams. If a women's team has to leave the weight room when a men's team comes in, you have a problem. If the men are kicking women off the lifting stations, you have a problem. At many schools there are times some sports need to share a weight room, but the scheduling needs to be done without regard to gender. Scheduling must be equitable and as convenient for one gender as for the other.

- Coaching—The gender equity folks are also looking for equity among staff members and checking whether members are certified and how they are assigned to sports or locations. They look at staff in terms of years of coaching experience of those assigned to men's sports versus those assigned to women's sports. They compare salaries of staff assigned to women's sports to those of staff assigned to men's.

- Weight room facilities—There must be enough quality space to accommodate teams without crowding. When athletes are interviewed, they sometimes report a perceived difference in treatment. For example, if female softball players perceive that football players are getting better treatment when they go to the weight room, you might have a gender equity problem.

Title IX has had a tremendous impact on sports conditioning. Women have gone from not being allowed in the weight room, not being allowed to eat at the training table, and not being provided travel and accommodations for competitions, to equal access to all these things and equal opportunities to improve performance.

Women in the NSCA

When I set up the bylaws of the NSCA in 1978, I made sure women were treated on a professional basis equal to that of men. The Augusta National, where the Masters' tournament is held each year, has received national attention for not allowing female members. That practice is very rare today, but in the 1970s it was much more common. I ensured that in matters regarding the strength coaches association that women had an equal voice. Kathy Calder was the first female member of the NSCA. She was the only female out of 76 members to attend the first NSCA convention. Jane Lilyhorn was the first national women's director in 1978 but resigned when she and I were married in 1979.

Karen Knortz was the first chair of the NSCA research committee. Meg Ritchie was the first regional director of the NSCA and the first female head strength coach in Division I. Meg told me she was influenced by John Anderson, the national track coach in Scotland. After seeing Meg compete in high school invitational track meets, Coach Anderson motivated her to pursue track beyond high school. Frank Dick followed Coach Anderson as the national track coach for Scotland and motivated Meg to pursue an interest in strength coaching. Frank is currently the chair for the European Track Coaches Association. Meg was motivated to get stronger after watching the great Russian thrower Fiana Melnik training in the weight room. Melnik bench pressed 380 pounds for four sets of four reps in 1973. Although Meg was one of the strongest women in the world herself, she was impressed by Melnik's achievement. Meg could bench press 350 pounds and clean 352 pounds. To get an idea of how strong these women were, consider that Thressa Thompson, a three-time national shot-put champion, cleaned 253 pounds for the Nebraska school record.

Meg was hired by Cedric Dempsey, the athletic director at Arizona, as the first full-time female strength coach in history. Shortly after the Arizona Wildcats won the College World Series in baseball, Meg called us to discuss her baseball lifting program. She knew our reputation for strength training and wanted to compare notes. We spoke for an hour and never discussed any details of her baseball lifting program. I surprised her by telling her that the lifting program was secondary to motivating her athletes. I knew she had a solid lifting program, so I completely ignored it and discussed things I thought might help her improve the motivation and promotion of her program. I wanted her to see a much broader picture.

No matter what gender or sport you're working with, if you can convince players and coaches that your strength-training program is the best, they'll use it, and great results will follow. The mind controls the body, and one of the keys to success is to motivate the athletes to train hard for long periods at high intensities when it's no longer fun to do so. Many athletes, especially younger ones, need positive proof that strength training will benefit them before they're willing to put forth the effort needed to obtain maximum results. They need to *believe* in the program.

The key is to get athletes to want to achieve new goals. Once they begin achieving goals, they'll be eager to set higher goals. It's always better to pull back on an athlete who is motivated rather than one who needs to be pushed. When starting a lifting program, purposely keep the weights light for the first few weeks. The first week, athletes will feel a sense of accomplishment just by finishing the workouts. The next week, they'll focus on the prescribed poundages used. If the prescribed weight is too great, your athletes will struggle and burn out in a few weeks. By keeping the prescribed weights lighter, you'll keep the carrot out there for them to reach for. They'll gain confidence as they complete the second week's workouts and be hungry to add weight the next week. Software packages are available to help strength coaches prescribe poundage systematically over time. Remember that it's where your athletes end up that counts, not where they start out.

If you're looking for a new way to motivate your athletes, try writing a weekly newsletter that promotes hard work and brings attention to athletes who perform at a high level. Regularly updating school records and awarding T-shirts for certain levels of achievement are also good motivators.

All of this is what I talked to Meg about when she called to talk about our lifting program at Nebraska. Yes, an excellent lifting program is important, but many other areas are important, too. A great strength-training program means little if you don't get your athletes to buy into it. Incidentally, Meg Richie is now Meg Stone. She married Dr. Michael Stone, one of the top strength researchers in history, and she is considered one of the best strength coaches in the country.

Influence of the Strength Coach

In the 1972 Summer Olympics, Russian sprinter Valeri Borzov created quite a stir with his success in the 100 meters. Many in the United States thought Borzov was either on drugs or had a secret scientific approach superior to anything seen in the United States. But what really led Borzov to excellence was a systematic lifting program. Through his achievements, Borzov demonstrated that athletes could no longer rely on natural size and strength. Soon after his success in the Olympics, strength coaches sprang up around the United States, dispelling the notion that strength training is incompatible with running, swimming, track, and other non-contact sports.

Athletes began training year–round, adhering to programs that changed in the off-season, preseason, and in-season. This new focus on training created a new term, "periodization," which hadn't been used much before by sports coaches. Coaches in the United States now have sophisticated, computerized programs that help produce great athletic performances. Lifting weights has become accepted by society and has even worked its way into TV commercials as a method of obtaining a positive image. Just 30 years ago, commercials made fun of people who lifted weights. They were considered geeks. Today, superstars such as Michael Jordan and Tiger Woods are known for their work ethic in preparing their bodies for competition and training with weights. Strength training has completely turned the corner and is accepted as a positive way to improve performance, boost confidence and self-esteem, and promote overall fitness.

All of this success means strength coaches now have a far-reaching influence over players and coaches alike. Sports Illustrated writer Tim Layden describes strength coaches as being "second only to the head coach—a close second—in the influence they hold over the players and the role they play in steering a program toward a national championship" (1998). He describes the various roles that strength coaches play in athletes' lives, including those of "trainers, dietitians, spies, counselors, and surrogate parents" and likens their office to a confessional. While only 30 years ago the profession didn't even exist, today strength coaches are considered absolutely vital to a program's success.

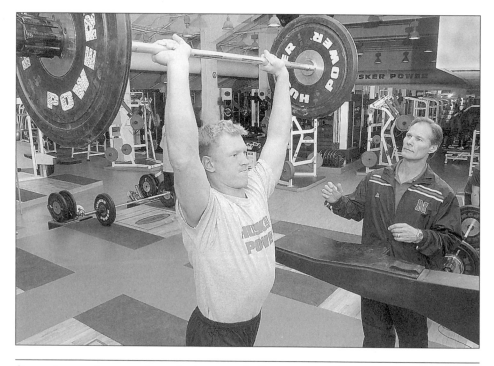

Strength coaches now have just as much, if not more, influence on athletes as head coaches, helping them achieve success both in and out of the weight room.

Steroid Use in Sport

East Germany led in the development of a sports culture to produce champion athletes, but in the process the athlete has often become an experimental subject. The East Germans spent enormous amounts of money to identify athletic talent in children and develop high-quality coaches and specialized training routines. Behind the East German operation was the systematic doping of athletes. The worldwide sports community had a fear in the late 1960s and early 1970s that Eastern European and Soviet bloc countries were going to dominate the athletic scene with their apparently superior athletic training methods. As it turned out, this was a time of much experimentation and mystery concerning drugs—both legal and illegal—with scientific labs that were later discovered to have developed a whole new generation of drugs designed to promote growth and sport performance. The American College of Sports Medicine (ACSM) claimed that steroids did little, if anything, to enhance athletic ability. But athletes knew better because their experience had demonstrated otherwise. The NCAA banned performance-enhancing substances in 1973. Before 1973, these drugs had been legally distributed and lawfully consumed by athletes who needed only a doctor's prescription to get them. Strength coaches at that time usually had backgrounds in weightlifting, powerlifting, or bodybuilding. These early strength coaches sometimes bowed to the pressure of permitting steroids because their use had become commonplace. But after 1973, most strength coaches working with team sports in America took an antisteroid position.

Nebraska has always had to answer questions about steroid use because the Nebraska running game is a physical style of football where players tend to wear opponents down and dominate in the fourth quarter. But no athlete at Nebraska has ever been encouraged to use steroids. When rumors surfaced that some of his players were taking steroids in 1983, Tom Osborne asked his medical staff to institute drug testing immediately. He wasn't about to allow drug use, period. Back then, there weren't a lot of guidelines to go by. The testing was done, but it wasn't as sophisticated as it is today. For example, early drug-test procedures allowed athletes to be notified when they were going to be tested. When critics pointed out the drawbacks of this process, Coach Osborne changed to random, unannounced testing throughout the year. The Big Eight conference followed Coach Osborne's lead and initiated random drug testing the next year. Soon after, the NCAA began random drug testing at bowl games.

It wasn't until 1985 that the NSCA tried to tackle the steroid issue by supporting a scientifically based NSCA position paper and educational packet. Some programs still had their problems with steroids. In 1985, Doc Kreis pleaded guilty to one misdemeanor count of distributing a banned substance while at Vanderbilt University. He was able to put that behind him and has had a successful career at Middle Tennessee State and, later, as a master strength and conditioning coach at the University of Colorado and now at UCLA.

Oklahoma made headlines when it was one of the first schools to be reprimanded by the NCAA for using steroids. Three Oklahoma players were not allowed to play in the 1987 Orange Bowl game, including famed linebacker Brian Bosworth. That fall, the NCAA tested approximately 725 football players from 20 bowl teams. Of those tested, 21 players were found ineligible to play in their bowl games. In 1988, the University of Miami strength coach was suspended from the NSCA for a minimum of five years for a code of ethics violation regarding steroids. *Sports Illustrated* published an article in 1988 detailing steroid use within the football program at the University of South Carolina, and a year later their strength coach, Keith Kephart, pled guilty to a charge of transporting steroids across state lines. The NSCA was embarrassed because Kephart was a past president of the association.

In 1990, the NCAA expanded their required random drug-testing program to include other sports. The use of steroids by college athletes was reduced considerably by the NCAA's drug-testing policies, but once the NFL started testing for steroids in 1989, steroid use came to a virtual halt. No longer was there incentive for college athletes to take steroids to prepare for the NFL. If caught using steroids by the NFL, they would lose the opportunity to play in the league and get a big paycheck. As a result, steroid use in college is now a nonfactor. It's rarely seen today. Over the last 30 years, athletes have moved from viewing steroids as supervitamins to understanding that they are illegal substances that can ruin a good career.

Major League Baseball (MLB) is a different story and has been in a world of its own regarding steroid use. Until August of 2002, the baseball players' union did not have drug testing, and there was rampant steroid use in professional baseball. Unlike the NFL, NBA, NCAA, and the Olympics, baseball did no drug testing of its players. The issue of drug use in baseball made headlines when Mark McGwire admitted to using the legal steroid androstenedione in 1998, the year he broke the 37-year-old home run record held by Roger Maris. A reporter had seen the drug in McGwire's locker and asked him about it. Androstenedione was and is available over the counter because it's considered a food supplement. It comes from a natural source—tree bark. Even so, androstenedione use is banned by the NFL, NBA, NCAA, and the Olympics. Baseball will eventually curb drug use through testing. In 2003, the commissioner banned products with ephedrine for Minor League players. Once they can get the Major League players union on board, they'll progress to building lean body mass through strength training, as athletes in other sports are doing.

Many remember when Ben Johnson ran 100 meters in 9.79 seconds, the fastest 100 meters ever run. His effort in front of 70,000 people in the

Olympic Games in September 1988 broke the existing world record of 9.83 seconds. One day later, he tested positive for steroids, and Johnson was stripped of his record and gold medal. Because of the positive drug test, many people fail to recognize the benefits of the strength training Johnson did. Instead, they attribute all of his speed improvement to the drugs he used. He squatted 660 pounds in training leading up to the meet. Yes, the illegal steroids allowed him to gain the lean muscle mass, but the strength training allowed him to apply the force against the ground and increase his speed to run the fastest 100 meters in history. If you take drugs out of the equation, Ben Johnson showed how to develop speed. Coaches need to convince athletes that lean body mass and speed can be developed through strength training. Athletes need to understand that training, not drugs, is the key to success. Drugs aren't worth the risk to an athlete's health or reputation.

Side Effects of Steroids

Heart and liver damage

Increased risk of cardiovascular disease

Increased risk of liver disease and cancer

Increased risk of kidney disease

Increased risk of cervical and endometrial cancer

Feminine characteristics in men (breast enlargement)

Testicular atrophy

Masculine characteristics in women (deepening of the voice, irreversible increase in facial and body hair, decreased breast size)

Increased risk of osteoporosis in women

Irreversible enlargement of the clitoris

Amenorrhea

Uterine atrophy

Acne

Baldness

Aggressiveness

Decreased sex drive

Impotence

Infertility

Depression

Mood swings

Psychosis

Mental addiction

Athletes are getting bigger, and training is more sophisticated. Researchers have helped identify more efficient ways to improve performance. Women athletes are here to stay in athletics. Strength coaches have become a valuable part of athletics, and steroids are becoming a rare thing on the college scene. All of these things have helped shape the landscape of sports conditioning in the past 30 years.

2

The Path to Husker Power and Beyond

No one could believe athletes could actually gain 30 or 40 pounds and yet run faster. What Nebraska was doing made national news. Testing the players before and after the season provided me with the facts I needed to change attitudes toward sports conditioning for athletes. Our Husker Power program has been imitated by many in the last 34 years, but I'm proud to say our program is still recognized and trusted as one of the best.

My Introduction to Weightlifting

Many events contributed to the path to athletic power that is now Husker Power, including my first experience with a set of barbells. I discovered then that guidelines for athletes who wished to start lifting weights were badly needed. In 1957, when I was in fifth grade, doctors determined I had asthma and advised my parents to move from Nebraska to Phoenix, Arizona. While walking to school my first day in Phoenix, I met a classmate named Danny Lundberg, who proved to be a big influence on me and on the development of Husker Power. After a few weeks of school, Danny invited me and another boy named Ronnie Wilson over to his house. Danny took us out to his father's garage, where his older brother kept a set of weights.

This was Ronnie's and my introduction to weightlifting and likely resembled the experience of many other youngsters. The bar had 75 pounds on it at the time, and Danny was eager to demonstrate how he could clean this bar first to his chest and then over his head.

Without stretching, warming up with a lighter weight, or giving a second thought to proper lifting technique, I gave it a try, too. Peer pressure can be strong at age 10. The lift wasn't easy, but I managed to get the bar over my head and return it to the floor, much to Danny's approval. Now it was Ronnie's turn. Ronnie wasn't the athletic type, and I was worried for him because I knew how hard the lift had been for me. Ronnie managed to lift the bar to his chest, but when he jerked it over his head he lost control of the bar. He fell over backward, and the bar nearly landed on his head. From that little lesson, I quickly understood there was some technique involved with the sport of weightlifting and that lifting should not be done without knowing the proper procedures or having some supervision.

My next experience with weightlifting came in seventh grade when my parents surprised me with my own 110-pound barbell set. The York Barbell

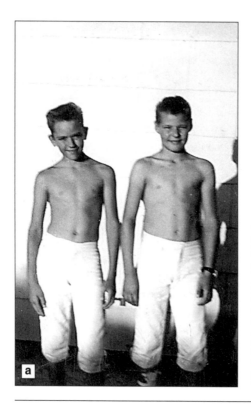 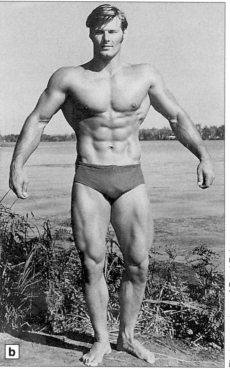

Photos courtesy of Boyd Epley

Before and after: *(a)* Danny and me when we first discovered weightlifting in 1957, and *(b)* me as a bodybuilder in 1972.

set came with instructions based entirely on competitive weightlifting. No instructions were included on how to improve athletic performance, and I didn't realize then that most coaches didn't recommend weightlifting for athletes. After the novelty of the new barbell set wore off, it began collecting dust. There was no recommended program for athletes to follow, so I lost enthusiasm. Other interests took over, and I didn't give lifting another thought until the summer after my junior year in high school.

In the summer of 1964, I became friends with Pat Neve, a bodybuilder my age who eventually became Mr. America and Mr. USA. Pat was very serious about his exercise routine and did arm curls during TV commercials. He would occasionally drag me along to a friend's house to train with him. Pat's friend, Ken Cole, was a teacher and coach at a grade school in Phoenix. Ken had a sophisticated set of equipment in his backyard where he let weightlifters and bodybuilders train.

I wasn't really interested in competitive weightlifting, powerlifting, or bodybuilding at the time, but I did want to gain weight and get stronger for football and track. Rather than impose on Ken, I joined a local health club where I could work out regularly. During that summer I combined some of the bodybuilding and weightlifting concepts with my own ideas and integrated some running drills to prepare for my senior football season.

My progress that summer seemed more dramatic than it would be for someone beginning a sports conditioning program today. It was like being the only person in town who had watered his lawn the entire summer. My "lawn" was noticeably greener and healthier than anyone else's on the team. It's hard to imagine such a situation occurring today because most athletes are lifting weights in their summer training programs.

People sometimes ask me, "What did bigger muscles and added strength mean to you?" I reply in one word: "Confidence." Lifting weights that summer started a chain of events that changed my life completely.

Gaining Confidence,
Strength, and Determination

My physical progress made me more disciplined and more dedicated to keeping a schedule. I became serious about anything that would help me become a better athlete. I watched what I ate for the first time, went to bed early, and tried not to miss any workouts. I was becoming an athlete and was anxious to show the results.

I had gained 20 pounds over the summer, so my football coaches moved me from quarterback to linebacker. Much to the surprise of everyone, with my new confidence, new strength, and new determination, I was able to set a school record for most tackles and was named the outstanding defensive player of the year. My success in the weight room gave me the confidence and strength I needed to succeed on the field.

My hard work had paid off, but it was only the beginning. I continued to lift weights and used my new strength to set records as a pole-vaulter. I won the Outstanding Track Man award for my high school. Some bad luck followed, however. I broke my leg just before the state championships, which kept me out of the state meet and spoiled my chances for a scholarship from Arizona State.

I directed my energies to pole-vaulting at Phoenix Junior College. I started as a "walk-on" but was granted a scholarship after I placed fourth in the national junior college track meet as a freshman. Perhaps because of my own experience, I have always had a deep respect for the athletes who come to Nebraska as walk-ons. Many demonstrate a work ethic that earns them a scholarship down the road.

Ron Easton, the Phoenix College wrestling coach, was at a track meet and overheard me complaining. I was on the runway about to take my third jump in the pole-vault. I was complaining about how the wind was blowing in my face and how I couldn't get my grip right and if I missed the height I would be out of the competition. Overhearing me, Coach Easton told me something that has affected me every day since. He told me, "The great ones adjust."

Coach Easton was right. The wind was basically the same for all the vaulters, and the ones who could adjust would be the most successful. I made the height and went on to win the competition, but more important was the confidence those words brought me. Those four simple words released my anxiety and allowed me to focus. Those simple words have gotten me through some pretty tough situations since. They apply to nearly every situation. The great ones adjust. I have the words posted in the strength complex office at Nebraska, and the staff has heard them many times.

When I was a sophomore, the strength training continued to pay off. I earned a scholarship to the University of Nebraska after tying the National Junior College pole-vault record at 15 feet, 1-1/4 inches. My great uncle Howard Morris lived in Lincoln, Nebraska, and had coffee with the head track coach, Frank Sevigne, on occasion. He mentioned my success to Coach Sevigne, who indicated he would contact me when the Nebraska track team went to Arizona that spring to compete against Arizona State. After receiving a letter from Sevigne letting me know he would be in town, I arranged to have a practice session at the Arizona State track at the same time the Nebraska team would be working out. It was a very windy day, and the Nebraska and ASU vaulters were having a tough time with the wind. But I was having a great day. I was the only one over the bar at 15 feet that day, and Coach Sevigne approached me, extended his hand, and said, "Do you have an interest in Nebraska?" I said, "Yes." He said, "I'll send you the papers." I received the scholarship papers in the mail a few days later.

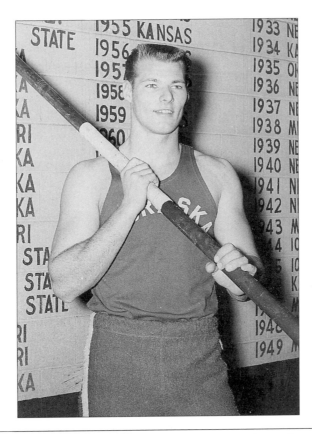

Weightlifting gave me the strength to set records as a pole-vaulter and earn a scholarship to the University of Nebraska.

Bringing Strength Conditioning to Nebraska

When I left Arizona after 10 years, I had outgrown my asthma problem and picked up a basic knowledge of weightlifting, powerlifting, and bodybuilding. I had no idea I would later take parts from each and apply them to what would be known as sports conditioning. I didn't realize it at the time, but I ended up helping to bring sports conditioning to Nebraska.

Arriving in Lincoln and making my first trip to the weight room, I had never seen such huge athletes with massive arms and legs. These gigantic bodies wandered into the weight room with no idea of how to train, and not one of them could bench press 300 pounds.

My extra strength enabled me to set the Nebraska school vaulting record, but it wasn't until I sustained a back injury that sports conditioning took over as my main goal in life. I went to the Husker weight room several times a week to rehab my injured back. There were a few other injured athletes in the weight room, but they didn't seem to know what to do, so they started following me around, trying out my exercise routine. At that time Nebraska athletes had no stretching program; no winter strength or conditioning program; no summer strength program; no testing of strength, agility, or power; and no lifting during the season.

As the 1969 school year started, I was supposed to be a senior pole-vaulter, but because of my back injury my track coaches decided to red-shirt me. This meant I would have a year to train before my senior vaulting season began. The extra year allowed me to spend much more time in the weight room. At the time, lifting was not recommended for healthy athletes, so those who wandered into the Nebraska weight room had some type of injury. One of the injured athletes was a star I-Back named Joe Orduna, who had just had knee surgery. Back then, arthroscopic surgery was nonexistent, and your career was normally over after you had knee surgery. Joe's lifting program helped him not only recover but play great football again; in fact, he was drafted in the second round by the San Francisco 49ers.

I learned that conditioning for football is similar to conditioning for pole-vaulting. Football players run 40-yard sprints and play explosive bursts in a game with the added resistance of a uniform. The 115- to 120-foot approach for pole-vaulting is a 40-yard sprint with the added resistance of carrying a pole. Both sports require athletes to be lean, strong, and explosive. When they saw that I was under 180 pounds but was stronger than most of them, the Nebraska football players started doing the program I had developed for myself. The players had little if any lifting experience, and they didn't have a structured program, so I filled a need for them. Other players also overcame their injuries via trips to the weight room, and one day I got a call from Dr. Tom Osborne, assistant football coach for Nebraska.

The Call From Osborne

I recall the conversation this way. Coach Osborne asked me if I was the guy who was showing the players how to lift weights, and when I said I was, he invited me to come to his office to talk about it. I thought I was in deep trouble. Coach Osborne had noticed how the injured players were coming back to practice with more development than before they were hurt. Osborne asked if I would be willing to work with the football team. If I could do this for the injured players, surely it would benefit the healthy ones as well, maybe even more. I seriously considered helping the football team, but I also knew my time at Nebraska as an athlete was winding down. I told him that I was just a student and had one more year to compete, but I would help as much as I could. I told him the weight room was so small that we could fit only 10 to 12 players in there at once. At that time, Nebraska had only one bench-press bench, a single bar with 390 pounds of weights, an incline board, a Universal Gym machine, and five dumbbells. The room was 424 square feet.

Coach Osborne said he could have a wall removed to enlarge the size of the room but would need help determining what equipment to purchase. He asked if I could make a list of what Nebraska would need to buy. There was an 8-foot-by-12-foot window on the west wall of the north fieldhouse that had been painted over so that coaches could show films in a classroom adjacent to the lifting space. The classroom was 920 square feet, so once the wall between was removed, we had a rectangular space of 1,344 square feet for lifting. It wasn't long before the 1,500-square-foot locker room adjacent on the south became available, and the north fieldhouse weight room was expanded to 2,844 square feet.

I brought Coach Osborne a list of equipment. I wasn't sure what his limit was, so I included the basic items needed for the football team to begin training.

Original Equipment List

Two squat racks and bars, lifting plates, and plate racks to hold them

One bench and bar, lifting plates, and plate racks to hold them

A light pulley system for shoulder work

Dumbbells in pairs from 5 to 100 pounds

Preacher curl bench and weights

Two work benches

Two seated incline benches

I also wanted to create an arm and shoulder area but wasn't sure Coach Osborne would go that far. I went ahead and listed some equipment just in case he might approve it. Coach Osborne looked at the list briefly then handed it to the football secretary with instructions to order everything. After seeing how easy it was to get the list approved, I quickly added, "Coach, I forgot to bring the other page." Osborne laughed and gave me a wink. He suggested I bring in the second page the following day. Well, I came back with the second list the next day, and I've been bringing lists ever since. Osborne looked at the second list, which included about half as much equipment as the first page, and asked, "Now, you're sure this is all?" After I nodded, he gave the additional page to the secretary to order. With space allocated and equipment ordered, the beginnings of a strength program were in place. But one big obstacle remained—getting the head coach to buy in.

Additional Equipment List

Fixed barbells

E-Z curl bars

Neck machine

Lat pull-down

Low lat pull

Coach Osborne told me we needed to visit with Bob Devaney. Bob was the head football coach and athletic director at Nebraska, and he was beloved by all Big Red fans. We went into Coach Devaney's office, where he was sitting behind his desk.

Coach Osborne explained to Coach Devaney that he thought it would be a good idea to have the entire football team start lifting weights. Coach Devaney asked, "Why?" Coach Osborne introduced me and explained how I had been showing the injured football players how to lift. These injured players were coming back to practice much stronger. Coach Osborne predicted, "If the injured players increased their strength levels, healthy players should get even more benefits. Lifting weights could turn our football program around."

Coach Devaney was skeptical. He said he didn't know of any other football programs lifting weights. His good friend Duffy Daugherty at Michigan State didn't have a lifting program. On the other hand, Nebraska had finished their last two seasons with 6 and 4 records. They were looking for

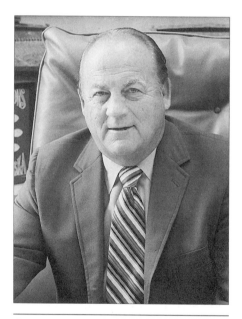

Coach Devaney's words to me before I helped implement a lifting program for football players: "If anyone gets slower, you're fired."

something to give them an advantage over other teams. Tom Osborne was an intelligent and innovative coach, and Devaney thought highly of him. He finally went along with the idea but with some reservations. "I won't make the lifting program mandatory. The players can do it if they want to," he said. Then he looked directly at me and added, "If anyone gets slower, you're fired." He didn't know I hadn't even been hired yet.

But the prospect of a job came just at the right time. That same week, the Nebraska team doctors determined that my back injury was not going to allow me to compete in pole-vaulting any longer. My career as an athlete was over. The idea of becoming an employee of the athletic department, initiating a strength program and supervising the weight room, was appealing but challenging.

First Paid Strength Coach Position

On August 15, 1969, Nebraska became the first school in the Big Eight Conference with an official strength coach. Many of the football players had never lifted before. In the early days, working with them was a little

When I'm asked who influenced me to start Husker Power, I respond, "My mom and dad, for starters." My dad was a roofing contractor, so I never really learned to work by the hour. When I could, I helped my dad and older brother roof on weekends. We worked until the job was done. Over my years as a strength coach, the work ethic I learned from my father has paid big dividends. My parents also saw the physical changes and confidence that strength training had given me, and they encouraged me to pursue strength training as a career.

Another big influence was my pole-vault coach at Nebraska, Dean Brittenham. Coach Brittenham and I had a great relationship, and I considered him my early mentor in athletics. Tom Osborne was my mentor for 25 years thereafter. Coach Brittenham has two sons who are strength coaches in the NBA. He encouraged me to stay in college and get a masters degree so I could continue coaching on the college level. I asked my college instructors at Nebraska if I could gear my coursework toward learning more about sports conditioning programs and facilities for athletes. They were great and let me tailor most of the classes around the strength-coaching job I was doing for the athletic department.

like standing on an interstate trying to get all the traffic to stop, turn around, and go the other direction without getting run over. Fortunately, Nebraska had recruited three California junior-college football players, Dick Rupert, Bob Newton, and Keith Wortman, and one from Phoenix named Carl Johnson. All four had lifted weights and helped set a good example for the others. These four made it much easier to get the program off the ground.

With Coach Devaney's words ("If anyone gets slower, you're fired") echoing in my mind, I decided to find a way to show him that his players could get stronger, bigger, and faster all at the same time. Unfortunately, this would be tough to prove because there weren't many resources available. Athletes weren't being tested at the time. In addition to borrowing stopwatches from the physical education department chairman, Dr. Carl Wear, I also asked if he knew of any tests that were good indicators of talent. Dr. Wear mentioned that the jump-reach (later to be called the vertical jump) might be a good indicator of talent, although it had not been used much. I included the vertical jump in my battery of tests. I also asked the physical education department to allow me to create lifting classes that the football players could take for credit. This would allow the best opportunity for athletes to focus on lifting within a controlled environment, both in the in-season and the off-season. The PE department agreed, and lifting classes were initiated soon thereafter.

I tested the football players on the 40-yard dash and a few other tests before and after the season, and then tested again just before spring football. Much to the surprise of everyone but me, all the players gained muscle, and they all got faster. Today it's common knowledge that athletes can gain 30 or 40 pounds or more and yet run faster. But at that time, this was big news.

Changing Attitudes Toward Strength Conditioning

We didn't win our first game of the 1969 season against USC, but we gave a great effort and surprised a few people around the nation by coming back in the fourth quarter and giving a strong Trojan team a good scare.

Nebraska's first football win after the initiation of the Husker Power program occurred on September 27, 1969, in the second game of the season, when we beat Texas A&M 14–0. Nebraska finished the 1969 season with nine wins and beat rival Oklahoma 44–14 in Norman—at the time, the worst loss ever for Oklahoma on their home field. What a dramatic turnaround from the 47–0 home loss Nebraska had suffered to Oklahoma on national television the year before they started lifting. Word of Nebraska's strength spread quickly around the country. Meanwhile, Nebraska athletes pounded their opponents that year, including a 45–6 defeat of Georgia in the Sun Bowl.

Most of Nebraska's improvement in the win–loss column in 1969 came as a result of young Tom Osborne's brilliant play calling, but I got to keep my job, too. Everyone agreed that our new strength program was a success. In fact, my salary tripled from $1,000 to $3,000 per year. Over the four years after adding the lifting program, Devaney's record at Nebraska was 42–4. When he retired after the 1972 season, he had the winningest record of any active coach. Later, he was inducted into college football's hall of fame.

I was just a graduate assistant for my first two years with the Nebraska football team, and the strength program was barely underway, but schools were starting to visit Lincoln to see for themselves what I was doing right, and it wasn't long before they were hiring away my assistants. Meanwhile, Nebraska had opened many eyes across the country by winning back-to-back national championships in 1970 and 1971.

Attitudes were changing toward strength training. Track and football athletes were the first to get started lifting. Then one day the basketball coach, Joe Ciprano, stopped by and asked for a lifting program for his players. Joe wasn't sure about lifting, but some of the powerhouse basketball programs had started lifting programs and were seeing the benefits. Swimming was next to start lifting, and baseball followed soon after.

Expanding the Program
for More Men's and Women's Sports

With more and more sports using our lifting facilities, I wanted to add a circuit training area, but I didn't have enough space. Finally, in 1973, I was able to add the circuit room in the south stadium. Initially, I relied on football graduate assistants to supervise the room for an hour each day. John Sanders, the baseball coach, came to supervise his own players, which helped a great deal.

In 1975, we added 10 women's sports all at once. They all wanted lifting programs, so in 1978, we added the Bob Devaney Sports Center Weight Room, where most of the female athletes trained. In the early days of strength training for women, coaches and athletes didn't want to train with iron because they were afraid the athletes might get huge muscles. Instead, they used isokinetic machines we ordered for them. But isokinetic machines give only the perception of explosive action. The harder you push, the more the machines resist. They actually slow down the movement as you try to accelerate through the range of motion. It didn't take long for the women's coaches to realize that the $20,000 worth of isokinetic equipment we put in for them didn't produce the strength, speed, and agility they were expecting. Soon afterward, they were asking to convert to free weights.

Bernard Cahill was a Cybex salesman I enjoyed talking philosophy with. He understood what I was after probably better than anyone else, even though he was selling Isokinetic units. Bernard's units were not going to get the job done for athletes, but he helped me form beliefs in free-weight principles that I still hold today. Free weights still make up the base exercises at Nebraska (the squat and clean have always been the basic lifts), and machines are used for supplemental exercises and circuit training. The circuit programs have changed a little over the years, but they still have their place for muscular endurance. We got away from the squat for a few years when I developed the hip sled for American Manufacturing Foundry (AMF). It took us a few years to discover that there's really no substitute for the squat, and we gradually replaced hip sleds with more squat racks.

The Emergence of a New Profession

Prior to 1977, there was some confusion about whether strength coaches were allowed to travel with football teams or to stretch athletes at away games. Strength coaches were not considered part of the football staff, and anything they did was subject to debate. Jim Williams, my first assistant,

Since coaches Tom Osborne and Bob Devaney asked me to start the sports conditioning program at Nebraska, we have had 20 national team championships in volleyball, gymnastics, bowling, and football. The five national titles in football have gained Nebraska's strength, conditioning, and nutrition program national recognition as the premier program in the nation. As head football coach, Tom Osborne won 255 games and three national championships in 25 years. During my first 33 years, every Nebraska football team won at least nine games and each year played in a bowl game. The 2003 Alamo Bowl in San Antonio, a win over Michigan State in which we held the Spartans without a touchdown, extended this NCAA record to 35 straight bowl games. One of the most impressive feats over this 35-year period is that every football player who came to Nebraska for four years won at least one championship ring.

recalls, "My first two years at Arkansas I was not allowed to travel with the football team, so I had to travel with the alumni group in order to be at the away games to stretch the team. My next two years I was allowed to travel, but only after Jimmy Johnson (head football coach) and Dean Weber (trainer) requested permission for me to do so." Some schools had strength coaches traveling with the team, and some schools did not even have a strength coach, which prompted the NCAA's first legislation restricting strength coaches' activity. In January 1980, the NCAA repealed the rule that prohibited strength and conditioning coaches from participating in stretching and warming up athletes for any varsity sport. Strength coaches were finally recognized for their contributions, and NCAA rules started to make more sense for strength coaches.

As a result of a lobbying effort by strength coaches around the country, the 1991 NCAA legislation finally permitted voluntary training time. NCAA legislation was amended to permit unlimited, voluntary training time under the supervision of the strength and conditioning staff. This was a big turn-around for strength coaches, who just 11 years earlier were not allowed even to stretch their teams.

In 1974, Mike Arthur became the first paid assistant strength coach at Nebraska, and he still remains loyal to the Huskers. Mike came to the weight room as a high school athlete from Lincoln East High School and showed a tremendous work ethic, so I let him train in our facility. I thought maybe his work ethic would motivate some of our athletes. Rules at the time didn't allow high school athletes to train at a university unless they were enrolled in a camp. By the time he was 16, Mike Arthur was the strongest person in the state at 132 pounds. He won the state powerlifting title 10 straight years in addition to the national championship. In April of

1976, when Mike was a junior at Nebraska, I was the faculty advisor and coach of the UNL weightlifting and powerlifting teams. I asked Mike to be coach, even though he was only a junior. Mike won the 1977 National AAU Collegiate Powerlifting Championship and the 1977 Junior National Powerlifting Championship. Over a 10-year period, Mike was in the top five best powerlifters in the world at 132 pounds. He retired from lifting after setting a world-record deadlift of 540-1/4 pounds. He gave up powerlifting and wrestling to dedicate his time to a career in strength coaching.

I realized early on that Mike's tremendous work ethic in the weight room carried over to everything he did, so I asked him to help me while he was still in college. At first, Mike wasn't paid, and for years he didn't get to travel with the team or go to bowl games or receive many of the perks that other coaches did. Fortunately, those things were never important to Mike. He asked for an opportunity to do research in the strength field,

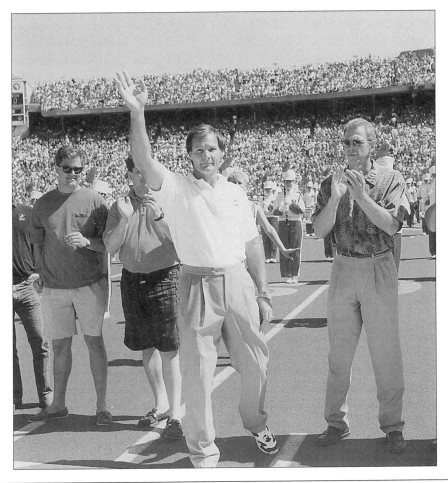

The Nebraska College Hall of Fame rewarded my loyalty to the Husker Power Program by honoring me at Memorial Stadium in 1993.

In 1976, Rick Forzano of the Detroit Lions offered me the opportunity to be their strength coach. At the time, only the Pittsburgh Steelers, Dallas Cowboys, Houston Oilers, and San Diego Chargers had strength coaches. At first I said yes to the Lions' offer, but Tom Osborne talked me into staying with the Huskers. He told me, "Their coaching staff could all be fired next year, and you'll be out of a job. If you stay with me, I'll be there for you." That's all I needed to hear. Tom was right—the entire Lions staff was fired the next year. Meanwhile, at Nebraska we continued to average 10 wins a season. In 1978 we celebrated our 100th win since Husker Power was started with a victory over Penn State 42–17.

and for years he did just that. He has been a great partner for me through the years and provided stability in our program. His research has made a tremendous impact on the direction of the Husker Power program. In 1994, Mike was named assistant director of the Performance Team and director of the programs, which meant he took on more day-to-day duties of the program. Bryan Bailey, the coordinator of reconditioning, was reassigned to coordinate the strength research. In 1995, Mike was named National Strength and Conditioning Coach of the Year by the Professional Football Strength and Conditioning Society. In 2000, he was promoted to associate director of the program and took on even more of the day-to-day operation of the program for both winter and summer conditioning for football. In June of 2003, Mike was named director of athletic performance and took over most of the day-to-day operations for me for the 22 sports other than football.

During my 34 years as head strength coach at Nebraska, we lost 49 strength coaches to programs across the nation. Many programs have benefited from the Nebraska philosophy. Jim Williams was my first assistant but was hired away by Arkansas before he was even paid at Nebraska. The same happened with Donn Swanbom, who was hired by SMU, and Steve Bliss, who was hired by Miami. Both were hired before they were paid a salary. In the 1970s, phone calls from Woody Hayes, Barry Switzer, and other head coaches lured away my assistants one by one. The University of Miami hired me to develop their lifting facility, then hired Steve Bliss without even interviewing him just because he was from Nebraska. The New York Yankees, San Francisco Giants, Chicago White Sox, and California Angels all hired one of my assistants as well. Notre Dame and Florida State lead the list of acquiring the largest number of Nebraska assistants. Notre Dame has enticed three to come work for them over the years, and Florida State has three former Nebraska assistants currently on staff.

My path to athletic power began with my lifting introduction in Danny's garage. As I gained confidence in my strength improvement and found success in athletics, this led to a Nebraska scholarship. An injury changed the path and strength training began to grow and spread across the nation with Tom Osborne's support. Many athletes and coaches contributed to the direction the path has taken and many lives have been impacted.

3

Redefinition of the Athletic Body

A strength and conditioning program should be based on scientific principles. Too many times, coaches design programs based on the same drills their coach used. Others try to copy what the state or national champion is doing. Although it makes some sense to imitate what has worked for others, your primary basis for your strength and conditioning programs should be scientific principles that have been statistically proven to be effective.

The key to enhanced athletic performance is increased lean body mass, not a reduction of fat. The redefinition of the athletic body means increasing muscle. As athletes increase muscle, they will see an improvement of performance. Fitness-minded people training at health clubs are usually looking to lose fat. Their training involves a lot of aerobic work to burn calories so that they'll look better and feel better. A strength coach is less concerned about how athletes look. Their goal for their athletes is building lean body mass—putting a bigger engine on their frame so that their bodies produce more force against the ground to run faster and jump higher.

Performance Indicators

Dr. Chris Eskridge helps Nebraska's Performance Team regularly evaluate each component of Nebraska's conditioning program to ensure a sustained direct relationship with onfield performance. Chris looks for specific skills that correlate to actual field performance. For example, many years ago it was determined that the vertical jump had the highest correlation to onfield performance for power sports. Subsequently, athletes in power sports now commonly undergo conditioning programs to improve vertical jump performance.

Testing is done to identify correlations with athletes from all sports and positions, and conditioning programs are developed to address the onfield needs of the athletes in those sports and positions. Every few years, Dr. Eskridge and Mike Arthur reevaluate the conditioning program to ensure it's enhancing the skills necessary for onfield performance. For example, are the conditioning drills improving vertical jump performance? We also examine a range of skills to make sure they still highly correlate to onfield performance. The vertical jump continues to test out as the number one indicator of onfield performance for power sports.

Vertical jump index points are available on the huskerpower.com Web site. Go to the coaches menu option then Vertical Jump Calculator. Enter your weight and how high you jumped to calculate your vertical jump index points. A score of 500 is considered a solid performance for Division I athletes.

We separate strength tests from performance tests because strength tests are not good indicators of talent. Ironically, the improvement of strength increases muscle mass, which does improve performance. The increased muscle allows more points to be scored in the four performance indicator tests. Chapter 7 describes the tests used to measure performance and includes a chart of school record vertical jumps. The performance index points are explained in more detail in chapter 8.

If you're a coach who trains power athletes, you will want to look for athletes who can accelerate for short distances, have good lateral agility, and can jump high. Don't look for kids who can lift the most weight. Lifting hard likely indicates good work habits, but talent is what a coach needs to build a team. Once you locate talented athletes and get them to train hard, you have a winning combination.

Increasing Lean Body Mass

Our body composition research led us to discover that the key to enhanced athletic performance is not reduced body fat but increased lean body mass. This discovery made for a profound point of departure for our program and significantly influenced how we go about conditioning. Knowing that small gains in body fat won't adversely affect performance, we focus the core of our program on conditioning activities that increase the lean body mass of our athletes. We begin with teaching good lifting technique because this leads to strength development. Strength development improves lean body mass and also enhances the four performance indicators, which makes for improved performance on the field (see figure 3.1).

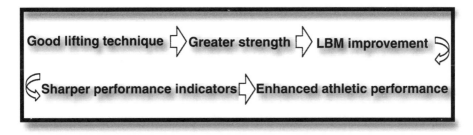

Figure 3.1 Performance improvement flow chart.

After discovering the benefits of lean body mass, Nebraska's Performance Team set out to find the most effective way to improve athletes in this area and thereby improve their performance indicators. This led us to employ the 10 core principles of conditioning outlined in chapter 4.

Our primary objective is building a base of muscular size. Scientific studies indicate that high-volume workouts build muscle mass, which increases the potential to build strength and power later. High repetitions alone are not the answer for athletes. This base phase (3 sets of 10 reps) builds mass and reduces body fat.

Unfortunately, many coaches believe aerobic conditioning prepares power-sport athletes for game endurance. But according to Dr. Michael Stone and Harold O'Bryant, among many others, building an aerobic base doesn't offer significant improvement in athletic performance for power sports (1987). Edward Fox and Donald Mathews proved power sports are anaerobic, not aerobic, activities (1971).

At one time, Nebraska collected an athlete's body composition data from seven sites (chest, triceps, scapular, AX (axilla), supra iliac, abdominals, and thigh) to calculate his or her percentage of body fat, which was quite time consuming. Consequently, after measurements taken on some 15,000 Division I athletes were reviewed, a new lean body formula was developed using only three sites. The three sites for men are the chest, abs, and thigh (figure 3.2). The three sites for women are the triceps, supra iliac, and thigh (figure 3.3). Our measurement process is now much faster and carries only an inconsequential validity error. The new method has proven to be most effective.

The key element in lean body mass computations is *consistency*. Although the three-site body composition test carries a high validity coefficient, it is extremely important to test athletes in the same way each time to ascertain changes in lean body mass.

A couple of examples come to mind of athletes with increased lean body mass that led to improved performance. Over one year, Husker offensive tackle Adam Treu gained 44 pounds of lean body mass, and softball pitcher Jenny Voss gained 12 pounds of lean body mass. Both athletes significantly improved performance in their sports (see tables 3.1 and 3.2).

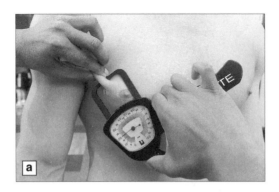

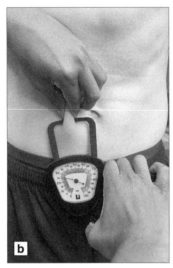

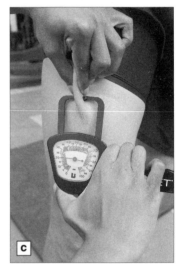

Figure 3.2 Three sites for men: *(a)* chest, *(b)* abs, and *(c)* thigh.

Table 3.1 Adam Treu's Improvement

Weight	Muscle	10-yard dash	40-yard dash	Pro agility run	Vertical jump (in.)
227	222	1.92 (E)	5.44 (E)	4.75 (E)	22.5
305	266	1.83 (E)	5.10 (E)	4.24 (E)	26.5
78	**44**	**-0.09**	**-0.34**	**-0.51**	**4.0**

Muscle Strength Versus Endurance

During strength training or short sprints, exercise is *anaerobic,* which means it's done without oxygen. A set or drill usually lasts only 15 to 30 seconds before a burning sensation is felt in the muscles. This burning

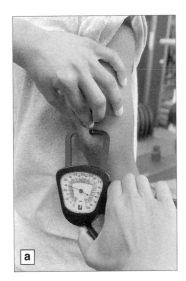
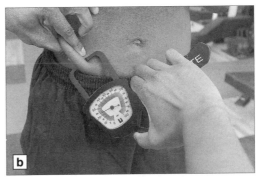
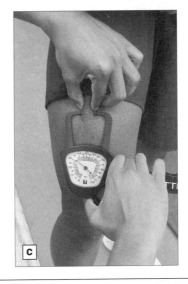

Figure 3.3 Three sites for women: *(a)* triceps, *(b)* supra iliac, and *(c)* thigh.

Table 3.2 Jenny Voss' Improvement					
Weight	Muscle	10-yard dash	40-yard dash	Pro agility run	Vertical jump (in.)
141	115	1.86 (E)	5.47 (E)	4.85 (E)	19.5
151	127	1.80 (E)	5.44 (E)	4.41 (E)	25
10	**12**	**-0.06**	**-0.03**	**-0.44**	**5.5**

is caused by a build-up of lactic acid, which is a waste product of adenosine triphosphate (ATP). When lactic acid build-up becomes too great, the muscle becomes fatigued to the point that it needs time to recover. During recovery, the body goes through a series of chemical reactions to supply more ATP. The amount of rest needed between lifting sets depends on the intensity of the exercise period and on whether the goal is increased strength or increased endurance. Resting one to two minutes between each set produces greater strength gains, whereas resting only 10 to 20 seconds between sets improves muscular endurance.

In general terms, there are two types of muscle fibers: slow twitch for endurance and fast twitch for speed. Everyone has a certain combination of slow- and fast-twitch fibers, which is determined at birth. Someone with a greater percentage of slow-twitch fibers can excel at endurance-type activities, such as distance running and swimming. Someone with a high percentage of fast-twitch fibers can succeed at sprinting and power-type athletics such as football, basketball, and baseball.

The recommended strength-training program will recruit more fast-twitch (speed) fibers but will not increase the number of these fibers—only the size. The speed fibers are able to contract faster and more powerfully than slow-twitch fibers do; they also increase in size and diameter to a greater extent as a result of strength training than do slow-twitch fibers. The larger speed fibers enable athletes to lift heavier weights. Distance runners don't have large muscles because they are recruiting slow-twitch muscle fibers when they run.

Muscles, and only muscles, can produce movement of the body. When you improve muscle strength, your movements become more efficient. You'll be able to run faster and jump higher, and you'll look better and feel better about yourself. This extra confidence should carry over into your everyday life.

Athletes in Weight Category Sports

If a wrestler wants to improve his performance but is afraid to add more muscle because doing so will increase his body weight, his best option is to lose fat. This allows him to increase muscle and perform at a higher level. Wrestlers perform best in an anabolic state. When wrestlers train to lose fat and increase muscle, rather than decrease muscle mass to make weight, they'll improve performance and have a higher level of energy during matches.

How Much Is Too Much?

Coaches are always concerned about their athletes' muscles getting too bulky, resulting in a loss of speed or mobility. In general, as athletes gain muscle they improve their speed, but at some point they might lose some mobility if they get too big.

You can usually recognize when an athlete is starting to gain too much weight to the point where it starts to hamper mobility or athleticism. For example, a football lineman might not be able to get out of his stance as quickly as he once could, or he might be unable to move with enough

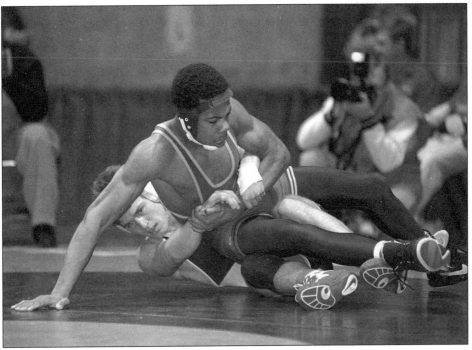

Athletes in weight category sports, like wrestlers, should train to lose fat and increase muscle, rather than decrease muscle mass in order to make weight.

speed and agility to reach his blocking assignment. A skilled-position player might become slower or less explosive or athletic. Usually when this occurs, it's a result of added fat, not muscle. In my opinion, you can never gain too much muscle. Muscle is functional tissue that helps athletes perform better. As long as athletes remain flexible and train correctly for their sport, the added muscle makes them faster, stronger, and more powerful. If you see a reduction in speed, strength, or power in one of your athletes, the added weight is probably not muscle mass. For the best exercises for gaining muscle mass, see chapter 11 for information on the squat, bench press, and incline press.

Look for athletes that can generate power, not ones that can lift the most weight. Have them train to increase lean body mass, which will make them stronger and more powerful. When you see an improvement in vertical jump, you'll see an improvement in performance.

4

Principles of Conditioning

Strength coaches, or whoever is in charge of the lifting program, might answer to a variety of bosses. Sometimes the sport coach or administrator might ask the strength coach to do something that doesn't seem to make good sense. Maybe they read something in the newspaper or saw something on television that put a wacky idea in their head. Or maybe they just want to try a new fad that other programs are trying. It seems there's always something new happening because everyone wants to discover a better way to do things.

A program based on scientific research eliminates the need to try all the new gimmicks that come along. A program based on proven facts and not on an overzealous marketing or advertising campaign will achieve much better long-term results, and the strength coach will be able to justify the program to parents, athletes, and administrators. No one should ask a strength coach to implement something the strength coach doesn't believe in.

There are only so many exercises that can be included in a program. Each exercise that is added must be better than an existing one. The same is true for the equipment used. It's fine for equipment in your facility to come from different companies, but if a piece of equipment doesn't contribute to the improvement of performance, replace it with something that does. The list of lifting exercises and the drills that you have chosen should be the best ones you know of for improving performance.

The 10 principles presented in this chapter, when applied correctly, will maximize physical development for athletes in power sports. The principles are based on scientific research, which has proven to be the foundation of the most effective way to train athletes for power sports.

We pointed out earlier that good technique and increased strength will increase lean body mass. Lean body mass improves the performance indicators, which lead to improved sport performance. With these facts in mind, research experts Mike Arthur and Bryan Bailey and I set out to find the most effective way to improve lean body mass and the four performance indicators. What we learned led to some drastic changes in the Nebraska strength program. We had to drop some exercises and tests that we discovered had little to do with improving performance so that we could focus on those that do.

Some coaches might want to skip ahead to chapter 11 for a look at the recommended program, but at this point you're better off staying here and studying the principles discussed in this chapter. You might not agree with everything you read, but that doesn't change the facts. If a coach is doing drills or lifts that don't meet the criteria of these 10 principles, they should make themselves justify what they're doing. They might be putting their athletes at risk. Coaches who aren't following these principles could find themselves working hard to climb the ladder of success only to find the ladder is leaning against the wrong wall.

Principle 1: Ground-Based Actions

Sport skills are almost always initiated by applying force with the feet against the ground. Newton's third law states, "For every action there is an equal and opposite reaction." What this means is that when an athlete exerts a force against the ground, it causes an equal and opposite reaction in the direction of movement propelling the athlete along the ground. Athletes should have their feet on the ground during the execution of the major lifts. Coaches should select lifting exercises that apply force with the feet against the ground, such as the squat, hang clean, or push jerk. The more force athletes can apply against the ground, the faster they'll run and the more effective they'll be in sport skills.

In 1993, the Hammer Strength Company sent me a double-incline machine to try (figure 4.1a). A couple of weeks later, they called to see how I liked it. I told them it was broken. The dealer told me they would repair it immediately and asked what was wrong with it. I told them it had a seat on it. The dealer said, "Sir, all of our machines have seats on them." I said, "That's what's wrong with your machines. They're made for health clubs and are good for fitness, but athletes need to be on their feet when they train; otherwise, there's little transfer to their sport."

It wasn't long before I got a call from the owner, Gary Jones, who invited me to the national factory where they developed a prototype machine now known as the Hammer Jammer (figure 4.1b). The company then trade-

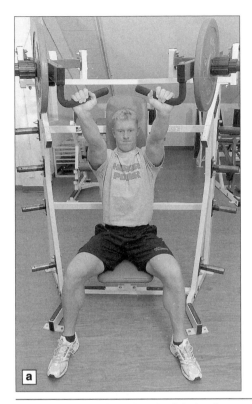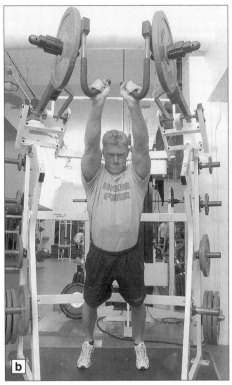

Figure 4.1 Unlike the double-incline machine *(a)*, the Hammer Jammer *(b)* allows for ground-based training.

marked the term Ground Base and began making other machines with no seats. This was the beginning of a focus on ground-based training that has spread across the country and led to many companies developing equipment on which athletes stand while performing an exercise.

With all the talk of ground-based exercises being superior, athletes and coaches were curious but not convinced. A simple illustration helped get Nebraska coaches and athletes to focus on ground-based exercises and drills. The strength staff asked their starting quarterback Gerry Gdowski to put a harness on, which raised him off the ground. Gerry was then asked to throw a football as far as he could. His best effort was 20 yards. We then lowered him to the ground, with the harness still on, and he threw 51.5 yards. This was definite proof that the use of his legs against the ground made a significant difference in his performance. We showed a videotape of this little test to the football coaches to get their help in convincing our athletes to focus on ground-based exercises.

The body's ability to stabilize joint actions contributes to proper neuromuscular coordination of the multiple-joint actions needed for most sport activities. The initial action of throwing the football originates from the muscular contractions of the hips and legs exerting a force from the ground in a backward direction. The earth, being more stable because of its large mass, doesn't move, and the reaction to this force is exerted through the athlete in a forward direction. As athletes extend their legs against the ground, their ankle, knee, and hip joints stabilize as the reaction force transfers to the torso. The torso rotates and then stabilizes as the muscular force is relayed to the chest and shoulders, and then to the arms and wrist, which displays the greatest motion. The force applied to the football is possible because the muscles effectively stabilize the joints as they sequentially contract. When Gerry was lifted off the ground, he couldn't throw as far because his leg and hip joints were not allowed to stabilize against the ground.

Coaches and athletes need to include the squat as a major exercise in their sports conditioning programs. Equipment companies continue to come out with new leg-press machines with features such as heavier weight stacks or independent weight stacks. But they are still machines you have to sit on. Consider these machines for fitness or, at best, for injured athletes. For healthy athletes who want to improve performance, there's no leg machine that substitutes for the squat. Unfortunately, if athletes are left to their own devices, they'll choose exercises that improve their appearance rather than those that improve performance.

Principle 2: Multiple-Joint Actions

Strength and conditioning programs should be based on exercises and drills involving multiple-joint actions to improve athletic performance. Two conditions must be met to be effective. First, each joint must be firmly stabilized, and second, the multiple-joint actions must be timed in the proper neuromuscular recruitment patterns. Training multiple joints will help develop coordination or the ability to generate explosive force. Training multiple joints will generate more force than training a single joint can. Isolating on single-joint actions might work for bodybuilders to improve their appearance, and it might work for rehabilitation from an injury, but athletes need activities involving multiple-joint actions so that a transfer of training in performance improvement occurs.

Single-joint exercises such as biceps curls, leg curls, or leg extensions contribute little to improve performance but are included in the program to build muscle mass and muscle balance. The recommended programs in this book are balanced to include at least one exercise for each major muscle group in the body.

Sport skills require multiple-joint actions timed in the proper neuromuscular recruitment patterns. Otherwise you have no coordination or ability to generate explosive force. Some people have natural coordination and will learn multiple-joint exercises, drills, or sport skills easily, whereas others will require coaching and disciplined effort to learn the correct techniques. Tiger Woods and Michael Jordan are examples of athletes with exceptional natural coordination. A video camera used to record lifting technique on the squat and hang clean might be the best instructor. Ask a certified strength coach to watch your form, and try to develop the best technique you can on these two major exercises.

Triple Extension

Figure 4.2a shows the acceleration phase of sprinting with the body positioned in a straight line and the ankle extended. When executed correctly, the body is also positioned in a straight line at the ankle position during a hang clean (figure 4.2b). During the extension, the body is positioned in a straight line at the ankles, knees, and hips. The summation of force generated by the triple extension is greater than any other force possible by the body.

Acceleration of a joint action is a key factor in the proper execution of sport movements (see figure 4.3). Most athletic movements involve a triple extension in which the force is generated in two or three 10ths of a second. Force is also generated on the hang clean and jammer extension in two or three 10ths of a second. The greater the force applied, the greater the acceleration.

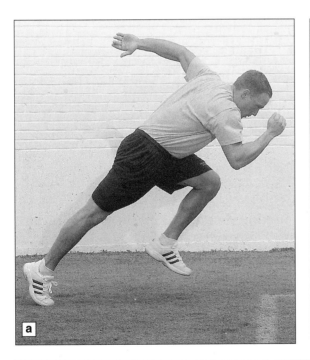 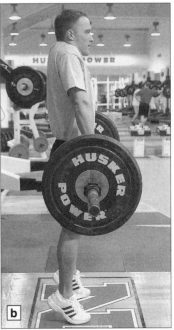

Figure 4.2 *(a)* The acceleration phase of sprinting is a straight line triple extension with the ankle extended. *(b)* The body is also positioned in a straight line triple extension during the hang clean.

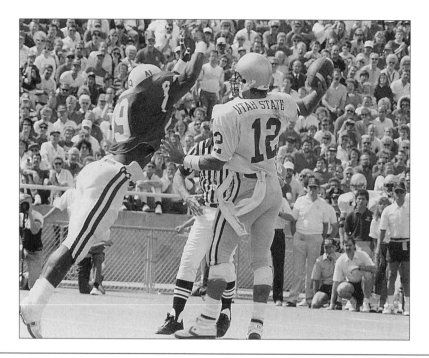

Figure 4.3 Here is an example of triple extension on the football field. The body is positioned in straight line triple extension to deliver maximum force.

Hang Clean Versus Power Clean

The body's ability to exert force depends on its position. The hang clean puts an athlete in the best leverage position to develop force, whereas the power clean from the ground can create problems for beginners. Some coaches have taught the power clean for years without any problems, but most would do better to teach the hang clean instead. Some beginners have trouble getting into proper leverage position when performing the power clean as they bring the bar from the ground to just above the knees. Teaching the hang clean allows beginners to learn how to execute the triple extension and generate maximum force. The power clean is done in the peak phase but only if proper form is accomplished with the hang clean in the development phase.

Picture an athlete in the "hit" position (see figure 4.4). From this position, movement is possible in any direction, whether the athlete is cutting to the left, hitting a golf ball, or spiking a volleyball.

When force is applied onto the ground, the athlete demonstrates a vertical jump. The vertical jump is a demonstration of the triple extension. Now try putting a light bar in the athlete's hand and having him or her do a vertical jump with the bar. This is called a clean shrug. The clean shrug is basically a triple extension with a bar in your hands. A hang clean is a

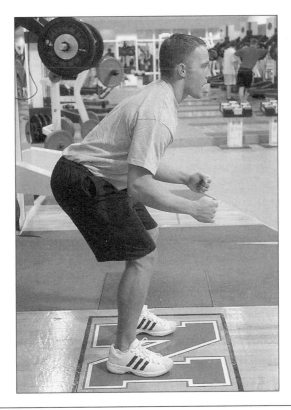

Figure 4.4   A body in the hit position is ready for triple extension in any direction.

clean shrug with the bar continuing on up to the chest. The hang clean then is a triple extension during which you catch the bar at chest level.

Strength Versus Power

One of the great advantages of the hang clean or power clean over most other exercises is their explosive nature. Most exercises require deceleration at the end of the movement, but these explosive lifts allow acceleration throughout the motion. For example, the squat is great for building strength, but you have to slow down at the end of the lift. You could jump off the ground to accelerate, but the weight would have to be extremely light to be able to perform the lift safely because you have to land with the weight. Gains would be minimal, and this is not a safe way to train.

Generally speaking, the squat builds strength, and the hang clean develops power. If velocity doesn't increase during the movement, acceleration is not possible. The recommended off-season program calls for two days a week focused on exercises building strength and two days a week focused on exercises developing explosive power. Only explosive lifts have transfer of training to sport movements.

Principle 3:
Three-Dimensional Movements

Sport skills involve movements in the three planes of space simultaneously—forward and backward, up and down, and side to side. Try to use free weights as much as possible in the selection of lifting exercises.

Strength programs should improve functional strength through exercises approximating these skills. Only free weights allow movement in three dimensions simultaneously. This makes the transfer of strength and power easier to merge with the development of sport skills. Machines limit the development of sport skills. For example, when you use free weights, the muscles regulate and coordinate the movement pattern of the resistance, while machines use lever arms, guide rods, and pulleys to dictate the path of the movement. Thus, machines limit the development of muscle synergism.

Synergism occurs when several muscles act together to produce a coordinated joint action. Only exercises using free weights allow synergism. The balancing action of synergistic muscles develops joint integrity better than machines do. For example, exercises using seats for support restrict the body from stabilizing properly; when doing leg presses, the adjustable board substitutes as the stabilizer, and the back and stomach muscles aren't required to stabilize the torso isometrically, as they would during the squat. When the torso is stabilized correctly, the body allows the legs and hips to work as a unit with the back and stomach muscles to perform the squat. The value carries over to the field or court when stability is needed to perform a sport skill.

The first casted selectorized weight stack and multistation machine was made in Germany in 1829, which means machines have been around a long time. But the only machines that come close to free weights for stabililty are the reciprocal push–pull machines developed in 2001 by Hammer Strength. These machines were developed at Nebraska to work both sides of the body and strengthen the core muscles in the torso while standing. In order for coordinated actions such as walking and running to occur, the body must use reciprocal movements. This means that one side of the body flexes as the opposite side extends. The push–pull machines use reciprocal movements to strengthen the entire body (see figure 4.5). As one side of the body extends or pushes the resistance on one side of the machine, the opposite side flexes or pulls the resistance on the other side of the machine. This strengthens the body in a way that is specific to the movements used when walking or running. Six push–pull machines make up a circuit program as outlined in chapter 11.

The last athlete I can think of who trained on machines only was Kelvin Clark in 1973. His high school in Odessa, Texas, had only a Universal Gym; consequently, he had very little stabilizer development when he arrived in Lincoln. His first day with free weights was an experience. Kelvin later developed into one of the strongest offensive linemen in Nebraska history. He once told me, "I was bench pressing 330 pounds on the Universal Gym in high school and thought I was pretty strong until I came to Nebraska and used free weights. I was shocked when I could bench only 260 pounds. I gained strength quickly, but I was in shock for a while."

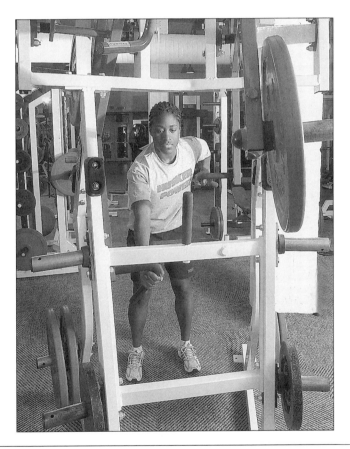

Figure 4.5 Hammer push–pull machines have unique reciprocal action.

Principle 4: Train Explosively

The amount of force required for a given activity is generally regulated by the use of two different types of motor units found in the body. Keeping this in general terms, you basically have fast-twitch and slow-twitch fibers in your muscles that vary greatly in their ability to generate force. Power-sport athletes are interested in developing fast-twitch fibers, whereas distance runners rely primarily on slow-twitch muscle fibers. You don't see many long-distance runners with bulging muscles. Their slow-twitch muscles rely on the oxygen system for muscular endurance, and not much strength or power is developed. Athletes who lift weights will develop their fast-twitch fibers, which means they can generate a force up to four times greater than a slow-twitch fiber, but not much endurance is developed.

The number of fibers a fast-twitch muscle fiber innervates is greater than with a slow-twitch fiber, and the contractile mechanism of fast-twitch muscle fiber is much larger. In most cases, power-sport athletes are born with a higher ratio of fast-twitch fibers, which allows them the natural potential to be powerful if they train correctly. There's a difference between being strong and being powerful. Athletes need to train for both.

Training explosively with free weights allows more fast-twitch muscle fibers to be recruited and in turn improves an athlete's performance potential. Athletes must concentrate to recruit the maximum force. There can be no horseplay in the weight room and no horseplay during competition. Athletes must learn to focus to recruit maximum force on each lift, drill, or play.

A motor unit is made up of a motor nerve and the group of muscle fibers that it attaches to. When a motor unit is stimulated, it will either contract fully or not at all. All contractions are of the same intensity because a muscle can't contract harder at one time than another. In a relaxed muscle, very few motor units are active. Just enough are stimulated at any one time to keep the body from collapsing. This is known as muscle tone. To lift a weight, it's necessary for the brain to call on more motor units to become active so the muscle can contract. The number of motor units that are activated is related to the amount of weight to be lifted, or the amount of weight you *think* you'll be lifting. The greater amount of weight lifted, the greater number of motor units activated to perform the lift.

If the force requirement is high and the athlete knows it, then a lot more motor units will be called on to do the job. Through training, the body learns to recruit more and more motor units so that more force can be generated and more poundage used. Sometimes the body is fooled into thinking the force will be high, and it's not. For example, if you tell someone to pick up a heavy suitcase that you have emptied beforehand, you'll have a demonstration of motor unit recruitment as they generate too much force to lift the empty suitcase they think is going to be heavy. During training, your brain determines how many motor units will be required to complete a task. A little variety in the training program keeps the body guessing and helps prevent a situation in which the brain sends only a few units to do the work that requires several. In a situation such as circuit training in which an athlete might use the same weight on each station over and over for several months, the body learns to recruit fewer motor units to do the work, and development is consequently limited.

Principle 5: Progressive Overload

Progression is defined as the act of moving forward toward a goal. The load, or amount of weight lifted, for each exercise is the most fundamental component of a strength-training program. Progressively increased loads make for continued improvement until the goal has been achieved. The application of the load has a crucial impact on maximizing performance and keeping injuries to a minimum. Overload occurs when the body responds to training loads greater than normal. The overload causes the muscle tissue of the body to go into a catabolic state or to break down. The body then adapts, through good nutrition and rest, by developing more strength or endurance to handle the overload.

Some coaches have added chains or bands to their lifts in an attempt to provide an overload during the lift. This is the opposite of what an athlete needs. To be explosive, we must train with acceleration throughout the movement. Adding a chain or band actually slows down the movement, and the movement gets harder as the bar is moved through the range of motion. That kind of training won't provide for the explosive overload needed in power sports. Recently, a high school coach told me of his state champion shot-putter who lost four feet on his throw during his freshman year at a university that was adding chains to his bench press. The shot-putter was forced to go back to his high school to train explosively in the summer to regain his former throwing distance.

Muscular strength is developed only when you use the overload principle. By applying the overload principle, you work your muscle beyond what's normal, and your muscle responds by adapting to the work imposed. Here is a summary of the adaptations that should take place as a result of our recommended strength-training program:

- Increase in number of motor units activated
- Increase in size of muscle fibers, especially the fast-twitch type
- Slight increase in capillary density
- Increase in strength of tendons
- Increase in density of bone at tendon attachment sites
- Increased ability of muscles to store ATP (adenosine triphosphate) for energy production
- Increased ability of muscles to tolerate lactic acid build-up

The novice to strength training will find strength improvements occur rapidly at first. Eventually, though, he or she reaches a point where progress stalls and improvement seems almost impossible. This is when a systematic approach that involves progressive increases is necessary to continue to produce good results.

Projected Max

When Nebraska wants to know the strength level of their athletes, we simply ask them to do a set for five or six repetitions. They then do a maximum effort with a weight they think they can lift for five or six reps. They might get 3 or 4, or they might get 7 or 8. If they get 10, we stop them. On most lifts, technique diminishes rapidly after 10 reps—plus, more than 10 reps measures muscular endurance, not strength. We have a computer in the weight room at all times for athletes to determine their one-repetition maximum (1RM). This method of determining 1RM is called a projected max. The athlete is not actually lifting the exact weight recorded as his or her 1RM but is lifting a poundage for a few repetitions that would equal the 1RM. All of Nebraska's school records are based on a projected max.

To determine your own projected max free of charge, go to the huskerpower.com Web site and select the coaches menu option, then "1 Rep Calculator." Some high schools have this site open during their maximum lift day to determine the projected max for their athletes. The problem with trying to determine strength levels or school records by just doing one repetition maximum is timing. Athletes might be strong enough to lift a certain poundage, but their timing might be off a bit, which causes them to barely miss their goal weight. It's difficult to assess then how much they might have lifted. We had that happen this past year when a lineman bench pressed 500 pounds for one repetition and then put on 540 pounds and missed it. He was probably capable of two repetitions at 500, which would have given him a 530-pound projected max, but instead he missed at 540 pounds, so no one knows what his actual strength level was.

Intensity

Intensity and volume are the key factors used to progressively increase the overload. The use of heavier loads increases the intensity. Adding more repetitions increases the volume. Each method causes specific adaptations. Increasing the weight and keeping the repetitions low develops strength and power. Increasing the number of repetitions and keeping the weight lighter brings improvement in endurance and muscular size. Strength coaches adjust the intensity and volume of the program to produce different results.

Intensity expresses the magnitude of maximum muscular effort. An intensity level of 100 percent equals the maximum load a person can lift for one repetition.

Intensity

75 percent (intensity) of 300 pounds (1RM) = .75 × 300 = 225

Use 225 pounds for your workout.

Volume

In strength training, the most common way to determine volume is by multiplying the number of sets by the number of repetitions to arrive at the total number of repetitions performed. This can be done for a single exercise, the entire workout, a week, a month, or a year.

Volume

Three sets of 10 repetitions is a volume of 30

Volume = (3 × 10) = 30

The volume of the training load plays an important role in the long-term planning of a strength program. Most studies indicate that muscular adaptations correlate to increases in volume. There's an inverse relationship between volume and intensity. The volume increases as the intensity of the load decreases. Excessive volume can cause a reduction in strength gains and eventually cause overtraining. One method our strength staff uses to monitor overtraining is the vertical jump. If the vertical jump goes down, we know the volume of training is too great.

Rest

Another factor used for overload adaptation in the recommended off-season programs is controlling the amount of rest between sets. A change in the amount of rest affects the training adaptation. Two or three minutes of rest between sets is normal in off-season programs using more than 70 percent intensity to produce muscle mass. Nebraska has shown incredible gains in muscle mass with its metabolic circuit, presented in chapter 10. By reducing the rest interval to one minute between sets and using intensities of 50 to 60 percent, gains that would normally take three or four years are made in four to six weeks. However, athletes can't maintain the intensity for more than six weeks. Using the same combination of sets and repetitions over an extended period causes strength to eventually plateau and diminish. The neuromuscular system grows accustomed to the same stimulus and becomes stale.

Principle 6: Application of Periodization

Untrained individuals respond favorably to most programs, thus making it difficult to evaluate the effects of different training programs for high school age athletes. Trained athletes show much slower rates of improvement. A review of Dr. Bill Kraemer's literature reveals that muscular strength increases approximately 40 percent in untrained athletes, 20 percent in moderately trained athletes, 16 percent in trained athletes, 10 percent in advanced athletes, and 2 percent in elite athletes over a period of up to two years (2002). This data shows a clear trend toward slower rates of progression with training experience. To bring about new gains, coaches need to change the repetitions and sets as the body adjusts to demands.

Seyle's General Adaptation Syndrome

Hans Seyle's general adaptation syndrome describes how the body adapts to training (see figure 4.6). If no variation occurs in the training stimulus, performance gradually levels off and overtraining follows. An approach to offset this problem is a system of training called periodization. Periodization adds variety to a program by using different combinations of intensity, volume, exercises, and drills throughout the training season. This helps avoid overtraining and stimulates peak performance. There are three distinct phases of adaptation to a strength-training program during the long-term application of the overload principle.

1. Alarm stage. This occurs during the first couple of weeks when starting a strength program. The muscles are in a mild state of shock, and muscle soreness occurs, along with a temporary decrease in strength as the muscles are forced to adapt. Poundage should be kept low for the first week or two to avoid making the muscles adjust too much.

2. Resistance stage. During this stage, the body begins to adapt to the stress of the strength program by growing stronger. The athlete makes good gains and feels good, and performance improves.

3. Exhaustion stage. Performance eventually plateaus and diminishes when the same strength and conditioning regimen is used over an extended period. If cycling is not done correctly, overtraining results and strength gradually levels off until eventually no progress is made. The neuromuscular system simply grows accustomed to the same stimulus and becomes stale.

Another example of Seyle's general adaptation syndrome occurs when swimming. At first the water seems cold (alarm stage), but after a few minutes the body adjusts, and the water temperature is comfortable

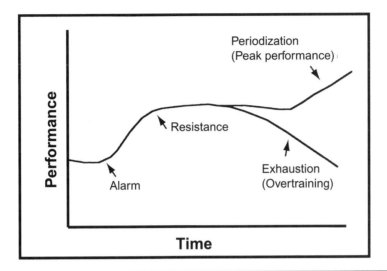

Figure 4.6   Seyle's general adaptation syndrome.

(resistance stage). After a while, the body can no longer fight off the cold (exhaustion stage), and the body can no longer tolerate the water. Once this occurs, it seems no matter what you do you can't get warm enough fast enough.

Periodization Phases

Strength coaches use periodization or cycling to permit continuous strength gains. Cycling progressively varies the training load, preventing strength gains from leveling off. In this program a cycle starts off with a base phase, which progresses to a strength phase and finishes with a peak phase. Phases are different combinations of volume and intensity, each translating into different responses by the body. Nebraska uses a pyramid to illustrate how much time to devote to each phase (figure 4.7).

The bottom of the pyramid, or the base phase, represents the greatest area or capacity of volume, whereas the top of the pyramid, or the peak phase, represents the least amount of volume done. More time is needed to develop the foundation or base phase. The height of the pyramid represents the magnitude of intensity. The program goes from high volume at low intensity to low volume at high intensity.

Base Phase

The primary objective of strength training is to build a base of muscular size. Scientific studies show high-volume workouts build muscle mass. Building muscle mass increases the potential to build greater strength and power later. This base phase also causes a reduction of body fat. Bodybuilders have developed very large muscles by doing high-volume

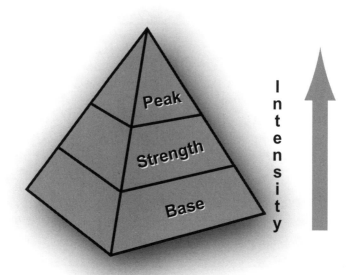

Figure 4.7 The Periodization Pyramid goes from high volume at low intensity to low volume at high intensity.

workouts with short rest intervals. However, high-volume workouts won't stimulate muscle growth unless the intensity is adequate. In the recommended program, the three sets of 10 have an average intensity of 70 percent with a volume of 30 repetitions. The muscle size increases through the process of tearing down and rebuilding muscle tissue. The lifting stresses individual muscle fibers and causes a breakdown. The body then adapts, and the muscle increases its cross-sectional size to meet the demands of future workouts. As the muscle increases in size, the athlete is able to handle greater loads in training. The muscle responds by growing larger again. There's a positive correlation between the cross-sectional size of a muscle and the amount of force it can apply. The larger the muscle fibers become through strength training, the greater their capacity to apply force. It's important to note that muscle size can only be accomplished by increasing the size, not the number, of muscle fibers. It's okay to include several single-joint exercises (leg curls, leg extensions, arm curls, and so on) in your program during this phase, but keep running to a minimum. Work large muscle group exercises before small muscle group exercises. Work multiple-joint exercises before single-joint exercises and do high-intensity exercises before low-intensity exercises.

Strength Phase

A strength phase calls for moderate volume and high intensity. Rest periods should allow the athlete to completely recover before attempting the next set. The amount of rest between sets and exercises significantly affects the metabolic, hormonal, and cardiovascular responses.

Longitudinal resistance training studies have shown greater strength increases with longer versus shorter rest periods between sets. Take two- to three-minute rests versus less than a minute of rest during this strength phase. The phase works best if it's preceded by several weeks of the base phase first. If you have 12 weeks to do a training program, have athletes do at least four or five of base phase (three sets of 10 repetitions) before changing to the strength phase (three sets of 5 repetitions). The strength phase has an average intensity of 80 percent. Athletes will need to increase the amount of weight used on the major lifts because they're doing only 5 repetitions instead of 10. By using more weight and lifting it for fewer reps, athletes will notice significant increases in strength. If you have more than 12 weeks to work, you might repeat the base and strength phases before moving on to the peak phase. Save the peak phase until two or three weeks before the season.

Peak Phase

This phase builds on the base and strength phases by developing explosive power, which is the combination of strength and speed. Volume is kept low in this phase, allowing athletes to lift poundage with speed. The three sets of 4, 3, and 2 have an average intensity of 85 percent with a total volume of nine repetitions (three sets of three repetitions). More power is produced when the same amount of work is completed in a shorter period of time, or when a greater amount of work is performed during the same period of time. A program consisting of movements with high power output using relatively light loads has been shown to be more effective for improving vertical jump ability than traditional strength training with heavy resistance. Heavy-resistance training might actually decrease power output unless accompanied by explosive movements. Although an 85-percent load is used for increasing the force component of power, a lighter 30 to 60 percent load can be used at an explosive velocity for increasing fast force production.

The lifting program should move from high volume and low intensity to low volume and high intensity. The hang clean, jammer, or push jerk are recommended because they've been shown to require rapid force production. Drop single-joint exercises during the peak phase to prevent overtraining.

Principle 7: Split Routine

Most fitness-training programs include three workouts a week on nonconsecutive days, such as on Monday, Wednesday, and Friday. This approach gives muscles a day of rest on the off-days before the program is repeated. In this program, muscles are worked three times a week.

In 1993, a few linemen asked to do a six-day split routine. Brendan Stai and Zach Wiegert, long-time NFL players, and Rob Zatechka, who gave up the NFL for medical school, called the six-day split routine the "real deal." They had three workouts, with workout 1 on Monday, workout 2 on Tuesday, and workout 3 on Wednesday. They then took Thursday as a recovery day before repeating the three workouts on Friday, Saturday, and Sunday. Monday then became a recovery day before three straight lifting days, and so on.

Most school systems wouldn't be able to consider a six-day lifting schedule—plus it requires a very disciplined athlete to stay with it. The offensive linemen were a big part of Milt Tenopir's famous "Pipeline" that helped produce a national rushing title and national championship in 1994 against Miami.

The "Real Deal"— Six Day Split Routine

Monday	Workout 1
Tuesday	Workout 2
Wednesday	Workout 3
Thursday	Rest
Friday	Workout 1
Saturday	Workout 2
Sunday	Workout 3
Monday	Rest

Modern sports conditioning programs use a much better program called a split routine. This is a very efficient and widely used principle in stimulating gains. Split routine simply means splitting the body parts and working them on alternate days. For example, you do half of the program on Monday and Thursday and the other half on Tuesday and Friday. The split routine allows half of the body to recover and rebuild while the other half is worked. The benefit of the split routine is that there are at least two full days of recovery before working a particular lift again. The split routine also allows athletes to include speed and agility drills without over-training. The program calls for speed and agility drills to be done before the strength workout. Train four days a week, working each lift twice, and allow at least two days of rest in between. Have your athletes take Wednesday off in addition to the weekend because their bodies will need time to recover. For many years now, Nebraska has closed the strength complex on Wednesdays to encourage athletes to recover properly. We take recovery for our athletes very seriously.

Principle 8: Hard–Easy System

One of the principles that's hard for many to understand is the hard–easy or heavy–medium principle. Most people believe that training as hard as possible every time is the key to greater strength gains. When athletes have a great work ethic, we figure they're working harder each and every workout. That would be a fast ticket to burnout. A great work ethic includes training smart, and that means training hard only on days you have scheduled to train hard. The fact is that athletes can make more progress over longer periods of time if they don't work at maximum loads during each workout.

The hard–easy system (table 4.1) helps eliminate overtraining and mental burnout. With this system, there's only one hard workout per week per body part. The other days are light workouts. With only one heavy workout load a week per body part, the body is ready both physically and mentally as the loads become greater. One mistake coaches make is overloading their athletes with too much too early. It's better to have them focus on technique the first few weeks and gradually increase the load. The first two workout days of the week (Monday and Tuesday) should be hard days. Thursday and Friday should be the easy days.

Back off on the workouts by reducing the volume and intensity. On hard days, athletes do three sets; on easy days, they do two sets using the backoff phases. The hard day has a volume of 30 repetitions (three sets of 10) and an average intensity of 70 percent. The easy day has a reduced volume of 20 repetitions (two sets of 10) and an intensity of 65 percent.

Table 4.1 Hard–Easy System

Monday	Explosive lifts, back, biceps	Hard
Tuesday	Chest, shoulders, triceps, legs	Hard
Wednesday	Rest	
Thursday	Explosive lifts, back, biceps	Easy
Friday	Chest, shoulders, triceps, legs	Easy
Saturday	Rest	
Sunday	Rest	

Principle 9: Specificity of Training

The primary objective of conditioning is to improve the energy capacity of an athlete to improve his or her performance. Unfortunately, many coaches believe doing aerobic distance running in their conditioning program prepares athletes in power sports to sustain energy levels through the end of a game. Nebraska has a reputation for power football in the fourth quarter mainly because Nebraska players haven't done any aerobic running in years. They used to. In fact, until 1982 we ran a 1.5-mile run for time, just as many other schools still do. Then AMF developed a watch that sent a signal from the heart to a monitor worn on the wrist. I bought five of these watches and had our football players wear them during the winter conditioning program to see what was happening to their bodies during exercise. What we learned changed the way athletes train for football in most programs today. We discovered we had been training football players aerobically. We made fast changes to incorporate rest into drills, between drills, and between stations.

According to Dr. Michael Stone, building an aerobic base contributes little to the improvement of a football player's performance. This might seem controversial and hard to believe, but it's based on how the body works and how the body gets energy to perform work. If we look at how the body gets energy, we find that it's supplied to the muscles through the food we eat. But we can't use this food immediately—it must be broken down into adenosine triphosphate (ATP), which is the immediate energy source for all muscle contraction. ATP for muscle contraction is made accessible through the interaction of three energy systems that can be represented by a hydraulic model of three interconnected storage tanks.

ATP-PC (phosphate creatine) system. The first tank represents the ATP-PC energy system. ATP can be supplied and regulated to the muscle only via the tap from the first tank, which is regulated by nerve stimulation from the central nervous system. High-intensity, short-duration activities, such as the 40-yard dash or hang clean, are performed using energy supplied from the ATP energy system. The energy from this source can be supplied immediately, and the amount of force generated by muscle contraction is high. But the amount of energy readily available to muscle is limited. During high-intensity exercise, ATP is depleted within six seconds. If intense exercise is continued for more than six seconds, the energy needed is supplied from the second tank—the lactic acid energy system.

Lactic acid system. The release of energy supplied to the contractile mechanism is now slower because the opening of the outlet from the second tank is smaller. Thus, the amount of force generated is reduced. ATP from the second tank is released from the breakdown of glycogen in the absence of oxygen. Through this process, a metabolic by-product called lactic acid accumulates. The highest accumulation of lactic acid is reached during activities that last from one to three minutes. If the second tank is emptied, too much lactic acid accumulates in the muscle, which causes pain, resulting in a loss of coordination and force production, as often occurs at the end of a 400- or 800-meter race.

Oxygen system. The third tank represents the oxygen system. This system is more specific to the slow-twitch muscle fibers used during activities requiring endurance over a long duration at low intensity. The diameter of the outlet from the third tank is very small, reducing the flow of ATP even more and generating less force but providing for hours of contractions.

In a nutshell, that's how the energy systems function. The first step in setting up a conditioning program is to determine the major energy system used for an athlete's sport. If necessary, videotape a game and time how long athletes actually work versus how long they rest in between bouts of work. If we apply specificity to conditioning, this means athletes should train in the same way as they play in competition.

Fox and Mathews of Ohio State determined the energy system requirements for most sports years ago. The sport of football is not a long continuous activity. Each play involves an effort of 100-percent intensity for roughly five seconds. Between each play is an average of 50 seconds of rest, which includes timeouts and penalties. The demand for ATP is high during a play, and as the play ends, the ATP tank is almost drained. The energy tank refills to almost maximum capacity between plays, allowing maximum intensity for the next play. This is the part that some coaches fail to realize. The refilling of the ATP energy tank continues even into the fourth quarter. During a play, the first tank is emptied and refilled during the rest between plays. This process is repeated each play. Thus, the energy supplied during a football game is almost solely from the ATP energy system. So, why do we still have football coaches who run their players long distances? Some coaches say they understand distance running is not the correct energy system for power sports such as football and basketball, but they do it for mental toughness.

One day, the NCAA will require strength coaches to train athletes in the correct energy system. After the death of three athletes in the summer of 2002, ESPN did a special on summer conditioning that brought about some change but not enough. All coaches must learn what the appropriate energy system is for their sport and what drills train that system. This one change would go far toward protecting athletes from unnecessary risks.

If an athlete's success depends primarily on speed, power, and agility, why not incorporate a conditioning program with drills and activities that involve speed, power, and agility? The drills should be short and intense, simulating a real game. I've been speaking to groups for many years about eliminating distance running for athletes in power sports, but many coaches haven't gotten the message. We still have coaches out there taking shot-putters and running them a mile and a half for time. Drills should mimic the needs of the sport as closely as possible. If an athlete performs explosively, the drills should be done explosively. If athletes compete on hardwood floors, then train them on hardwood floors. The better you simulate real game conditions in training, the more transfer there will be to the sport.

Principle 10: Interval Training

Conditioning programs for power sports should be based on interval-training principles. Interval training is work or exercise followed by a prescribed interval of rest. The program should be adjusted based on the needs of the sport. For football, include a work-to-rest ratio of 1 to 10 with periods that are very intense for 3 to 8 seconds and rest periods lasting from 30 to 80 seconds. Baseball, volleyball, and other power sports need similar rest between drills for recovery. Basketball and soccer are dominated by the anaerobic energy system for activities that require high power output such as sprinting, jumping, boxing out defenders, and changing direction to accelerate and decelerate. Basketball and soccer have proven to be 60 to 75 percent anaerobic, depending on the style of play. The ATP-PC and lactic acid systems supply energy for high-intensity activities lasting up to 15 seconds and 2 minutes, respectively.

Conditioning for basketball and soccer should incorporate drills and activities that train these energy systems. Recovery occurs during stops in play such as timeouts, substitutions, and half-time. Up to 70 percent of ATP is replenished in 30 seconds and is almost completely replenished within 3 minutes. If explosive activities last only 3 to 5 seconds, basketball and soccer players have ample time to recover before their next burst of energy is required. Work-to-rest ratios of 1 to 3 and 1 to 5 are specific to the sport of basketball and soccer and should be used in the conditioning aspect of training. The intensity and duration of the drills should directly parallel a real game. Also be sure to allow gamelike rest periods between work intervals. The athletes will recover and repeat the drills with peak intensity. Table 4.2 shows an analysis of a randomly selected segment of one basketball player for one minute of official time. The activity of the segment is classified by intensity into one of three categories: high intensity (sprinting and jumping), medium intensity (shuffling, setting picks, running the floor), and low intensity (standing, walking, slow jogging). During this span there were two offensive possessions and one defensive session.

It took about two and a half minutes to run one minute of actual game time off of the clock. During this one minute of play there were 11 seconds of high-intensity activity alternated with 22 seconds of medium-intensity and 27 seconds of low-intensity activity. During the two and a half minutes, the player ran a total of 474 feet, and each segment of play lasted less than 30 seconds. Differing tempos of play might occur at various times of a

Table 4.2 Basketball Intensity

Elapsed time	Intensity	Activity
14 seconds	Low	Walks the ball upcourt
1 second	High	Cuts and passes the ball
4 seconds	Low	Jogs to a point along perimeter
4 seconds	Medium	Shuffles and sets a pick
3 seconds	High	Cuts to the basket for a lay-up
29 seconds	Rest	Waits for the ball to shoot a free throw
28 seconds	Rest	Substitutions
8 seconds	Medium	Runs back on defense
3 seconds	High	Denies opponent the ball
5 seconds	Low	Follows opponent and boxes out
4 seconds	High	Sprints and jumps to rebound the ball
10 seconds	Medium	Runs and passes ball upcourt
39 seconds	Rest	Teammate shoots first free throw
4 seconds	Low	Stands at midcourt waiting for second free throw

game, some at a higher tempo and some slower. Regardless of the tempo of play, the primary energy system used in basketball is the ATP-PC energy system (and occasionally the lactic acid system). The oxygen system is not called into play—thus, interval training is needed to condition for basketball and other power sports.

General Conditioning Stations

Nebraska uses two types of conditioning stations: general conditioning stations and sport-specific stations. General conditioning is sometimes referred to as "county fair" conditioning because stations are set up for athletes to move from one station to another. All athletes do the same drills as they rotate from station to station. One of the benefits of this type of training is the camaraderie formed as each group of athletes finishes at the same time. The general conditioning station concept can work for any sport. The stations include basic drills that would benefit any power-sport athlete. Athletes from a variety of sports can be mixed together, or groups can be limited to athletes from one sport. If you have a small group of athletes, have one coach rotate from station to station with them to complete the circuit of stations. If athletes are assigned to each station, at least one supervisor is needed at each station. Rotate the groups throughout the program so they don't always start at the same station. Nebraska uses six stations that last three minutes each to begin with, but the duration can be lengthened to as much as four minutes after several weeks. All stations have two minutes of rest between them to provide for recovery and water breaks. Athletes are told that they're permitted to recover between stations to allow for very explosive drills to be done at each station. When it's their turn, a 100-percent effort is expected each time.

A common training error of many conditioning programs is that rest intervals are too short. In fact, some coaches don't allow any rest at all between stations. If the rest period is too short, athletes won't have enough energy to meet the demands of their next maximum-intensity effort, which means force output is reduced. This problem is very common. Coaches who make rest intervals too short cause force to be reduced, and slow-twitch muscle fibers are trained instead of fast-twitch fibers. Athletes resort to pacing themselves so they can finish the program, and in the end they have developed endurance instead of explosive power.

Sport-Specific Stations

In 1990, Coach Osborne asked me to add more agility drills to our program. In doing so, we divided the team into four corners of the field for sport-specific stations. The players would stay in their corner and do specific drills for their position rather than doing the county fair general drills for the winter program. The football coaches liked the position-specific drills because they could mimic what they wanted players to do at their position. After we did sport-specific drills in the winter program for six weeks, the football coaches would do similar drills in spring football practices. My staff would again do sport-specific drills all summer, and the football coaches would use many of the drills to warm up players during fall practices.

We started to see a bunch of overuse injuries in the groin area. Initially, some coaches and trainers thought the squat was causing these injuries, but on closer review we discovered that several soccer athletes around the world suffer from the same injury, and they had never done squats. Cutting back on the number (250 days per year) of sport-specific drills reduced the overuse injuries. As a result, in 2000 the sport-specific drills were eliminated in the winter program and done only toward the end of the summer program. Another drawback of sport-specific drills is that the four corners don't finish at the same time. Because each corner is doing drills that pertain only to their needs, the drills vary considerably from one corner to another. Some team camaraderie is lost (though position pride is developed instead). Just as in the county fair stations, it's critical for rest to be built into the drills and between drills. If the group consists of 20 athletes, don't have them all run at the same time. Have two or three of them run, then two or three more. While a few are running, the rest are resting. This builds recovery time into the station and allows for intense effort by everyone. Another way to ensure intensity is to time athletes as they do the drill, or have them race each other. Timing works best with smaller groups, whereas racing works better with larger groups.

Common Program Questions

Some questions about the principles of conditioning come up repeatedly after speeches I give or in correspondence I receive over the Internet. Most of the questions are from high school coaches. Following are some of the kinds of questions I hear most frequently.

If you play your games on Fridays, what days would you lift in season?

If you play your games on Fridays, in-season lifting would be on Mondays and Wednesdays. If you don't like the recommended program, you could do a combined explosive and strength workout on each day. Monday would be the heavy day and Wednesday the lighter day. Do the explosive lifts first, followed by the strength lifts.

What percentage do you use in-season?

As a rule of thumb, 70 percent of max 1RM for three sets of five repetitions is the benchmark for maintaining strength and power in season. I recommend that you work up to the 70 percent. For example, in week one of your in-season program you should train at 60 percent of 1RM, followed by 65 percent in week two, and finally 70 percent in week three. Do it this way to prevent any additional soreness and fatigue that might hinder an athlete's performance during practice sessions. To avoid staleness, strength loss, and monotony during the season, you should incorporate an unloading week every fourth week. This is as simple as decreasing the poundage used to the 60-percent level for one week and then proceeding back to the 70-percent mark the following week.

I have a 12-year-old son beginning football this fall. When is it best to begin exposing kids to lifting?

Research indicates that the prepubescent athlete, male or female, who strength trains can obtain significant muscle strength. Research also shows that strength training might improve some aspects of motor performance. There are many myths surrounding strength training. Athletes have been told that lifting would make them muscle-bound, slow them down, and throw off their shots. These myths have prevented many athletes from enjoying the benefits of strength training. The fact is there is no faster way for an athlete to improve athletic performance than through a balanced strength-training program.

For many years, there was confusion over determining the right age to begin lifting for children. In August of 1985, eight major sports medicine groups met to prescribe guidelines for prepubescent strength training. The general consensus from this meeting was that strength training for prepubescent boys and girls can be started at any age. They concluded that strength training is safe for prepubescents providing they use the proper equipment and program and that they have proper instruction and supervision. The key factor is whether the child is mature enough to accept instruction. Our experience is that most children are ready by age 10.

The advantages of lifting are much greater than the disadvantages, yet there are still questions concerning the effects of early lifting on a child's body, both physically and psychologically. Although the primary reason for starting a strength-training program is usually to improve athletic ability, this should not be the primary goal in the first years of a youngster's training. The emphasis should be on developing discipline through forming habits of following the prescribed workouts. Bad habits are hard to break and can lead to keeping an athlete from reaching his or her maximum potential later. Pay special attention to mastering the techniques for each exercise and drill. Supervision of young athletes lifting weights is critical.

How do you know what percentage to use to get started lifting?

The answer depends on your training level, novice or experienced. If you're an inexperienced lifter, there's no need to worry about percentages or poundage charts. Find a weight that you can handle comfortably and use proper technique for the required sets and reps. If you're able to complete the workout with that weight, simply increase the resistance for the next workout. Progress slowly, keeping in mind that proper technique is the key.

For the experienced lifter, percentages become more important. Using the Husker Power Poundage Chart in the appendix, find the columns with the required sets and repetitions for the workout. Follow the columns down until you find the poundage you think you can accomplish. After completing the workout, you'll have a predicted 1RM. Record this 1RM in your workout log. If the poundage was easy, increase your 1RM the next workout. If the poundage was difficult and did not allow good technique, reduce the 1RM the next workout.

What are your thoughts on core training? Is Nebraska using it?

We have developed a line of six machines with Hammer Strength called the push–pull circuit, which develops the core. Reciprocal training while standing develops the core better than anything else we've tried. We've incorporated the push–pull circuit at the end of the strength day program twice a week and also during the in-season twice a week.

How can I increase my vertical jump?

Be sure to check your vertical jump points on our Web site huskerpower.com. Go to the coaches menu option and click on Vertical Jump Calculation to enter how high you jumped and what you weigh to compare yourself to our greatest vertical jumps.

When I began testing Nebraska athletes, it didn't take too long to realize there was a correlation between an increase in leg strength and how high an athlete could jump. This is almost always followed by an increase in sport performance and running speed. Strength is the cornerstone of power and thus should be the base from which you build your jump-development program.

To improve on the vertical jump, athletes must improve their lower body power, which allows them to generate the greatest amount of force in the shortest amount of time. Place special emphasis on the hips and thighs because they play an important role in jumping. Focus on the hang clean and squat for explosive power. Although strength training is the key to improving the vertical jump, one of the most commonly overlooked factors is that of practicing the vertical jump itself. Jumping develops explosive power by conditioning the neuromuscular system to respond with as much force as possible.

I'm a high school athlete. Can you give me a lifting program?

The NCAA rules prohibit us from sending athletes or coaches a program free, so we put as much information on our Web site huskerpower.com as possible. We use ground-based exercises using multiple joints and free weights whenever possible. Basically, we use a four-day split routine with two days of explosive lifting and two days of slow movements. Many athletes purchase a CD or manual from Husker Power. Nate Kolterman, an offensive lineman from Seward, Nebraska, bought a book when he was 12 years old and starting training to be a Husker. The problem with books is that athletes need to read them and then implement the program on their own, which can be tough.

How do I increase my running speed?

The ability to accelerate to top speed is essential for most athletes. The components needed to improve speed and acceleration are speed drills, good running mechanics, and strength training. The program also requires intensity and recovery. The objective of strength training is to strengthen the areas necessary to improve speed while reducing risk of injury. The fastest sprinters in the world can generate great force against the ground, which allows them to cover more ground with each stride. The squat is the best exercise to improve speed. It develops the strength to apply force into the ground.

Because it's ground based, uses multiple joints, and is done with free weights explosively, it fits into Nebraska's way of doing things.

What did you think of the supposed tie between athletic pubalgia and squats?

A case study done in 1999 hinted that some Nebraska players who had this injury placed the blame on the squat. They indicated they first noticed the pain in their groin doing squats. The fact is that there's no scientific proof that the squat has ever caused one of these injuries. Even our own chief ortho-pedic surgeon, Dr. Pat Clare, will tell you the injury is an overuse injury. This means the cutting, turning, twisting, starting, and stopping action that athletes perform have a lot to do with causing this injury. That's why you see European soccer players with the injury even though they've never done squats. The squat has no replacement in terms of value to an athlete who needs to gain weight or improve speed. When one of our athletes was found to have a groin injury like this he was restricted from squats to allow him to heal. Once restricted, development for that athlete was also restricted and, consequently, recovery took several months. During this period alternative ways to load the legs without stress to the back or groin were used. None of these exercises, however, have been able to replace the benefits of the squat.

Can you build speed and strength simultaneously?

Speed and strength can be developed simultaneously without doing any speed drills. Strength development is the key. Sprinting is a skill involving multiple-joint actions powered by muscle contractions. Force generated by muscles exert-ing a force against the ground causes movement of the body in an equal and opposite direction of the applied force. The best way to get faster is to develop the muscles' ability to generate more force. Muscles also coordinate multiple-joint actions. Speed improvement is a natural outcome if strength is developed using exercises that use ground-based, multiple-joint actions.

Are you asking if you can train by doing speed drills and lift to get stronger simultaneously? If so, the answer is yes, but this is not as effective as strength training alone. Speed drills are added to the program prior to the in-season, more for the conditioning effect than for the speed development. Most of the speed gains come from the strength gains and not from doing speed drills. When the speed drills are added to the program, a good strength foundation should already have been accomplished earlier in the year. Thus, condi-tioning becomes a priority and strength training a secondary consideration during the preseason. Earlier in the year, strength is the priority and condition-ing a distant second priority.

What exercise or drill improves quickness?

The ability to change directions quickly comes from the ability to apply force into the ground using the triple extension. When the hips, knees, and ankles extend together, we call this the triple extension. Force is generated by muscles exerting a force against the ground, causing movement of the body in the opposite direction of the force. The triple extension is developed with the rack clean, hang clean, power clean, jammer extension, or push press. These are all done in an explosive manner and will improve quickness.

What will help acceleration for the first 10 yards?

The first step in improving acceleration is to increase leg strength and power. To run faster, you must be able to apply more force against the ground. This allows you to increase your stride length (the distance covered with each step). Generally, as stride length increases, speed increases. Exercises such as the squat and the clean help to improve leg strength and power.

The second step in improving acceleration is to improve starting skills. Proper starting mechanics (foot and hand placement, forward lean, and so on) can significantly increase acceleration. Drills such as form starts and position starts should be incorporated into the running program to improve start skills and to help transfer the strength and power gains made in the weight room.

How much rest between speed workouts is recommended?

Optimal performance for speed development requires adequate rest. To improve speed, the recovery must fall in the correct energy system. This can be done through interval training. Drills need to be done with high intensity followed by recovery periods. Depending on the athlete's fitness level, the resting interval might range between 30 and 60 seconds. For example, if you're training 15 basketball players, you could break them into three groups of five. As the groups rotate, taking turns doing drills, one group is working while two groups are resting and replenishing energy stores. Work–rest intervals for football are 1 part work followed by 10 parts rest. If an intense drill lasts 5 seconds, the recovery period should be 50 seconds.

During very intense lifting exercise, dynamic muscle actions produce external work and use more metabolic energy than supplemental movements. As a result they also typically deplete phosphagens to a greater extent. For major explosive exercises, a 2- to 3-minute recovery period is needed.

In a split routine, how much less percentage should be done on easy days?

The workload on an "easy day" in a split routine can be reduced by manipulation of the volume or intensity. If the athlete wants to stay with the same number of sets on both the heavy and light day workout, then reduce intensity of the workout by 10 percent for the light day. A better way to be sure the workout is lighter is to reduce the volume. Do this by reducing the number of sets in a workout (for example, go from three sets of 10 on a hard day to two sets of 10 on an easy day).

What are your thoughts on the creatine monohydrate for young athletes?

Many young male athletes in high school want to gain weight. We think of using creatine as a last resort. First, the athlete should have been consistently following a well-designed resistance training program for more than a year. We want to see a commitment to the lifting program. Then if the athlete is still having trouble gaining weight, we would look at lifestyle issues concerning sleep and extra activities that might slow recovery, such as too much basketball or distance running. Next they would need to illustrate that they were truly attempting to eat four or five times per day following a healthy diet. After all of these conditions have been met, the young athlete would become a candidate for creatine.

Following the 10 principles will bring about the best possible opportunity for improved performance. Choose ground-based explosive exercises that are multiple joint and overload progressively as recommended. Add drills that are done in the correct energy system and allow the proper rest interval between drills.

5

Support and Supervision

The success of a strength and conditioning program depends on support from the athletic director and administration, including financial support and vision for program growth. This chapter describes how administrators and donors have impacted the Nebraska program and how other models are successful. You'll get a look at a recommended supervision structure and tips on how to motivate athletes without punishing them.

Athletic Director's Support

Typically, the university-level strength coach works for either the athletic director or the head football coach. When I was hired by Nebraska in 1969, Bob Devaney filled both these roles. As Devaney moved into his later years as athletic director, I worked both for him and for football coach Tom Osborne. When Bill Byrne replaced Devaney as athletic director in 1992, the strength coach position became a departmental position that oversaw strength and conditioning for all 23 sports and reported directly to the athletic director as assistant athletic director and director of athletic performance.

Our model at Nebraska is a little different from most, but it works for us. At a few schools in the country, the football program still has its own strength coach and its own weight room with no involvement with other sports. Ohio State, Penn State, and Oklahoma are all set up that way. Others have dual head strength coaches. Louisville and Texas Tech have a head strength coach for football and a head strength coach for basketball. Tennessee has separate departments for women and men, with one head strength coach for female athletes and another for male athletes. The female athletes are not allowed to use the men's facilities and vice versa. Texas operated that way until they merged their men's and women's strength-training needs under the direction of master strength coach and assistant athletic director Jeff Madden. Madden also oversees the training table operation in a model very similar to what Nebraska had prior to June 2003.

When a strength coach reports only to the football coach, one problem is a false sense of job security. Football coaches earn over a million dollars a year at major schools. In most cases they make more money than the athletic director or the president or chancellor of the university. When overseen by the football coach, things can seem rosy for the strength coach for a while, but more often than not, when the head football coach is replaced, the strength coach's position is in jeopardy, regardless of his or her expertise, years of experience, or success. In 2001, BYU replaced retiring football coach Lavelle Edwards, and Dr. Chuck Stiggins, the long-time strength coach, was replaced when a new football coach was hired. Regardless of Chuck's talent and status as a master strength coach, he was not protected by the athletic director because the new head football coach wanted to bring in his "own man." I have a real concern about the lack of job security in the strength-coaching profession, especially when one sport disrupts the entire athletic department strength services. The medical profession doesn't have this problem. You don't see a new football coach bringing in his own doctor or trainer. I hope the future presents better job security for strength coaches nationally. The key is having solid support from a strong athletic director. If you don't have the support of your athletic director, you're on a slippery slope.

Financial Support

In 1976, when the Detroit Lions offered me $19,000 to become their strength coach, my salary at Nebraska was $7,000. Tom Osborne asked Coach Devaney to help keep me in Lincoln, and Devaney said he'd give me $8,000. When Tom told me Devaney had approved $8,000, I said, "Okay, 7 and 8 is 15. I could stay for that." Then Tom said, "No, he said $8,000, period." But Tom didn't stop there. He went to the physical education department and arranged for me to coordinate the weight-training classes for students for an additional $3,000 in income. Even so, the combined salary of $11,000 didn't compare to what the Lions were offering. I still turned them down. I knew that if I stayed at Nebraska, I would always have Tom's support—not only with future salary but with growth of the program and facilities.

In 1978, I signed a consulting contract with AMF for a position that lasted 13 years. Fortunately, it's the policy of the University of Nebraska Board

In June of 2003, athletic director Steve Pederson asked me to take on the role of associate director for performance and facility development. With this new promotion, it was impossible for me to spend time with the athletes on the floor of the weight room. Steve tried to free up some time for me by shifting my training table and nutrition operation responsibilities to another associate. However, we still needed someone who could focus on the football players, be on the floor of the strength complex, motivate the players to lift, and keep the lifting principles intact. Over the previous nine years as assistant athletic director, I had found it difficult to be there for the players and relied on my staff to implement much of the strength program. I oversaw the strength program and staff for football but was also responsible for the strength coaches and programs for the other 22 sports, the training table, supplements for all sports, the equipment in the west stadium strength complex, the sports center weight room, the track weight room, Husker Power Club and Board of Directors activities, the huskerpower.com Web site, and the awards program for all. And now Steve was promoting me to add the operation of all athletic facilities.

My first thought was for Mike Arthur to focus on football directly. Mike had been there for me for 25 years and was taking on more and more of my strength-coaching duties as I focused more on administrative work. The problem was that Mike would now need to take on many of the administrative duties in addition to the strength-coaching duties as we promoted him to director of athletic performance.

This left master strength coach Bryan Bailey as the clear solution to supervise football strength and conditioning. Bryan is in his 18th year with Husker Power and the athletes really love him. He makes time for the athletes and is one of the best one-on-one supervisors we've ever had. Before all of this transpired, I visited with head football coach Frank Solich and assured him that I'd be there for him and Bryan with anything they needed. Frank could have asked for a different strength coach, but he knew right away that Bryan was the most logical choice with the existing structure that Mike Arthur and myself provided. Bryan could focus totally on the needs of the football players and Mike would handle all the other sports. I'd be there to support them both but would have time to help the athletic director.

Unfortunately, rumors began to spread, and many friends across the country were wondering what was going on. They thought maybe Coach Solich and I had had a big argument that led to my reassignment. Nothing like that happened. Actually, what started the changes was a meeting our athletic director, Steve Pederson, had with Harvey Pearlman, our chancellor. The chancellor gave Steve permission to

(continued)

(continued)

proceed on a very special project that Steve wanted me to oversee. How important can a building project be? Important enough for me to end my strength-coaching duties and assemble a facility team to make the $50 million dollar Tom and Nancy Osborne Athletic Complex a reality. I had mixed feelings about not having time to work with the athletes, but I couldn't resist the challenge Steve put in front of me. Steve announced my title change from assistant to associate athletic director in June of 2003, but he wasn't ready to announce the building project until November. During that period there was some confusion as to what I was doing.

Steve announced the project in November, initiating a fund raising campaign that had me fly to 17 cities in three days. This helped people understand what I had been working on since June. There were more changes to follow, however. On November 29th the athletic director fired head football coach Frank Solich and replaced him with Bill Callahan from the Oakland Raiders. Callahan in turn replaced most of the coaches involved with football including Bryan Bailey, the strength coach. In an article in the *Lincoln Journal Star* (January 25, 2004), Callahan said, "I made a change, and with all due respect to Bryan Bailey, I made that change for the betterment of our team. I wanted to retain Coach Bailey, because he does have expertise and value here. He's very well-respected by our team and players, and I wanted him to be a part of this program." Callahan's choice for the head football strength coach was my former assistant strength coach Dave Kennedy. Kennedy, from Omaha, had worked for me between 1982-88. He left Nebraska when Steve Pederson hired him at Ohio State. He joined Pederson at Pittsburgh and is now back home in Nebraska. Bailey was asked to remain as his assistant. Kennedy will do well at Nebraska. He has the support of the athletic director and head coach, which is essential to success.

of Regents to encourage university personnel to supplement their income through outside activities. This allowed me to stay with the Huskers.

In addition to financial support, it's also important to have the support you need to expand and develop your program. In 1981, Bob Devaney allowed me to move the original weight room from the north fieldhouse to a space under the west stadium. This move made Nebraska's new 13,300 square-foot weight room twice the size of any other in the country at the time. Oklahoma had a new 5,600 square-foot room, and Indiana had 6,400 square feet. Devaney provided $204,000 for painting and carpeting but wouldn't approve any money for new equipment. I went to Tom

Osborne and explained that we needed $60,000 for new equipment. Tom said, "I'll see what I can do." When I checked back a couple of weeks later, Tom said, "I got you $90,000." I said, "Coach, I only need $60,000." Tom said, "You need to refigure that," and gave me a wink. I refigured and, sure enough, the new total was $90,000. That's the kind of support the strength program received from Tom Osborne.

Another example of Tom Osborne's belief in the importance of our strength program came unexpectedly. During the 1970s and 1980s, Nebraska promoted two areas in recruiting new student athletes. The heads of the university's academic program and strength program were introduced at all functions and promoted heavily in publications. Tom made it clear that he believed in both programs and strongly supported them. When Dr. Ursula Walsh, the director of the academic program, left Nebraska in 1985 to work for the NCAA, Coach Osborne paid me a visit. "What do you need?" he asked. I wasn't expecting the visit or the question, but I quickly answered that I needed a secretary to help with all the paperwork.

Tom was sending me a message that he wanted me to have everything I needed to stay at Nebraska and that he would lend support in every area that he could. I learned to keep a short list of needs handy in case I ever heard that question again.

Whether you're at the high school, college, or pro level, as a strength coach you need to develop a great relationship with your athletic director. Everyone serves someone, and the better relationship you have with the one you're serving, the more success you'll have in the long term. The boss is either working with you or against you. If your boss is working against you, I advise moving to a different job. One way to build a good relationship is to be considerate of your boss's time by providing a rough draft of what you want with the basic facts provided. I always try to bring my boss a choice of solutions and not just present the problem. Be prepared. Schedule a meeting and bring the agenda. Be brief and to the point. You probably know more about your problem, what caused it, and what might solve it than your boss does. Giving him or her the facts allows an informed decision to be made. Keep your boss informed of any changes in the situation, good or bad, and you'll have his or her support for future projects. Regardless of where you are or the size of your program, here's a rule of thumb when it comes to asking your boss for something: If it doesn't help your program win, or help you educate (or, in college cases, if it doesn't help you recruit), then from your boss's perspective, you probably don't need it.

Provide the details for his or her signature with no hidden costs. Don't say you want to order something and expect your boss to look up how much it costs. Have a plan; make it easy for your boss to say yes. Remember—it's not how many ideas you have that matters but how many you put into action.

Community Support

The Husker Power strength and conditioning program would not exist as it is known today without the support of the administration and the fans in the state of Nebraska. Randy York of the *Rocky Mountain News* in Denver pointed out

There's absolutely no question that Nebraska is better at developing football players than any other program in the nation. No other school has the commitment from the administration Husker Power has, and no other school has the system for developing players Nebraska has. The crown jewel of Nebraska's facilities is not its stadium or its fieldhouse. The crown jewel is the weight room. It's officially called the West Stadium Strength Complex. The WSSC is a shining testament to conditioning. Here a man named Boyd Epley practices his trade better than any other conditioning coach in the world. It is Epley and that incredible weight room that allow Nebraska to transform 180-lb. Nebraska farm-boy walk-ons into 260-lb. major college behemoths. In 1973, Osborne's first year, the average Cornhusker weighed 199 lbs.; in 1983 it was 216; in 1993 it was 222; and the 2003 team averaged 238. Some of the athletes they get thought they would never go to a place like Nebraska, but they come in here and see this place and they're convinced this is the place for them to develop to their potential. It all adds up—the support of the state and the administration, the development of the athletes is unmatched by any major college team. To the delight of those strong people braving those strong winters in those strong farmhouses, nobody does it better.

Another view of the support Husker Power enjoys comes from writer Joe Soucheray:

It's entirely quaint and altogether understandable out here in the middle of absolutely nowhere that even the weight room performances for Nebraska athletes are reported in the newspapers as routinely as hog futures or state income tax revenues. A recruit better be serious about strength training if he wants to play for Nebraska. The weight room even has color balanced lighting so records can make the 6 o'clock news.

These writers have captured a glimpse of what's important in Nebraska. Nebraska fans simply are not going to let the program down. If they can help, they will. As the football season approaches, there's a countdown each day in the newspaper. This loyal support has spilled over to volleyball, baseball, basketball, soccer, and even bowling on the Husker campus. The interest translates into support by fans who want to see Nebraska be successful. It also translates into support from the administration to improve salaries and facilities, which helps keep Nebraska's good people in town.

Husker Power Club

The College Football Association was developed when Georgia and Oklahoma broke the existing television pact. In 1985, budgets got much tighter, and money for staff was very hard to come by. I asked Bob Devaney for an additional $4,000 in salary for Randy Gobel to keep him on staff. I had Mike Arthur as my top assistant but felt I also needed to add Randy. Bob said he didn't have the money but that I had permission to ask the women's athletic director, June Davis, for help. June was very supportive and appreciated all Randy had done for the department, but her budget was even tighter than the men's.

This led, a few months later, to the development of the Husker Power Club. I was flying back to Lincoln after giving a speech, and I must have looked depressed because a man named Jerry Dolson introduced himself and asked what was wrong. He was a Nebraska fan and could tell something was bothering me. I explained that money was a problem. I told him I was losing assistants, and the budget did not allow me to keep them. Jerry suggested starting a booster club with the intent of raising money to help keep the staff. It was a great idea and just what I needed to get the juices going again. The next day, I asked Bob Devaney for permission to create a fund at the UNL foundation to which donors could send money directly to support the strength program. The immediate goal was to raise at least $4,000 a year to keep Randy Gobel. After that, we wanted to raise enough money to add other strength staff as well. Bob Devaney didn't like the idea. First of all, he didn't want his strength coach bothering his donors. Any money raised would continue to go into a general fund. Money was tight throughout the athletic department, and as athletic director he would decide where to allocate the funds. This line of thinking is prevalent among athletic directors nationwide and is a cause for frustration for many strength coaches today.

At this point I was very discouraged. I had been working on this problem for months with no relief. In desperation, I placed a slip of paper on Bob's desk. On it was a phone number. I explained to Bob that all he had to do was call this number and a Husker Power Club account would be set up within the University Foundation. All they needed was his permission. Bob looked at me and said, "What happens if I don't make the call?" I reluctantly responded, "You'll be looking for a new strength coach." I knew it was risky talking to Bob Devaney like that, but I also knew that if I didn't, nothing would get done. Bob made the call and requested that an account be set up.

I then invited several businessmen to a meeting, and the Husker Power Board of Directors was born. They have been great advisors. Jerry Dolson has since passed away, but Doug Marolf, Lanny Fauss, and Gary Lortz continue to serve as members of the original board. I have since spoken to most groups in the state of Nebraska, including country clubs, dentists, doctors, bankers, farmers, engineers, and anyone else who would listen to a request to support Husker Power.

In the early stages, I felt pretty good about the booster club. Steve Pederson, our recruiting coordinator (and now Nebraska's athletic director), was a member of the Husker Power Club Board of Directors in the early years of its development. I felt that I had momentum, so I decided to stick my neck out one more time with Bob Devaney. I asked him for the mailing list of the Nebraska ticket holders. Devaney laughed and said, "I don't give that list to anyone." I pushed further by saying, "Probably because no one has ever asked you for it." Devaney laughed again and repeated that he didn't want me bothering his boosters, so I said, "You give me the list, and I'll have anyone you trust go through the list with a marker and cross off any name they recognize as a booster. The big boosters will not receive a letter." Bob relented and told me to ask Gary Fouraker, director of business and finance, to trim the list.

Gary Fouraker crossed off about 1,000 names that he knew were donors in addition to being ticket holders. To all the others, I had letters sent,

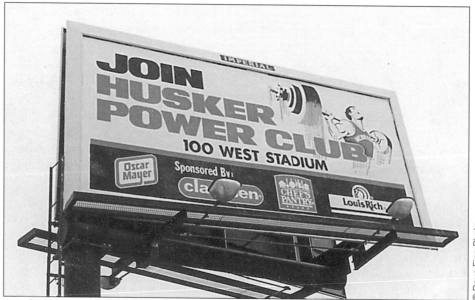

Husker Power Club promotional billboard.

© Dave Finn Photo

asking for $35 for a membership to the Husker Power Club. Over 800 fans responded to the mailing, which raised over $40,000. Bob Devaney was amazed at the support from the fans and their interest in helping the strength program. From then on, he was extremely supportive of everything I asked for. Somehow a light came on when he saw that fans were willing to support the strength program directly. The Husker Power Club was the first such strength program booster club in the country. Without Coach Devaney's support and vision, the program would not have an endowment fund from which interest is drawn each year to support the Nebraska strength and conditioning program and staff. What's really amazing is that nearly 300 of those initial 800 fans are still members of the Husker Power Club, having sent a donation each of the past 18 years.

In 1989, Devaney surpassed even Tom Osborne in his support of our program's strength-training facilities. When I proposed the weight room be expanded under the west stadium at a cost of around $800,000, Tom said, "The facility we have is fine." This time it was Devaney who pushed, telling Tom, "It will help your recruiting, and I think we should do it." By this point, their roles were reversed somewhat in that Osborne was now making the major decisions for the department, and Devaney had backed off into more of a consultant role. Osborne went along with Devaney's suggestion and told me, "We can provide $200,000 for the project, but you'll have to raise the rest." I gave Dan Cook of Dallas a call. Dan was a member of the Husker Power Club and had been instrumental in having an indoor field, aptly named the Cook Pavilion, constructed for Nebraska. I told Dan about the weight-room project.

"How much do you need?" he asked.

"$600,000," I told him.

"I'll give you $200,000," he said. "Meet me at the Waldorf Astoria Hotel in New York when we play Texas A&M in the Kickoff Classic in New Jersey, and I'll get you a check."

I recall renting a car for $29 in New Jersey where the team was staying and paying $60 to park the car near the famous New York hotel. When Dan saw me enter the room, he came over and said, "How much did I say I would donate?"

"$200,000," I replied, afraid the donation and the entire project was about to go down the drain.

Dan said, "How much do you still need?"

"$600,000."

"Just a minute—I want to talk to my wife, Gail. I'll be right back." When he returned, he said, "We want to donate $500,000 to your weight room."

How do I describe the joy of that moment? That donation changed my life in many ways. Dan and Gail will never know how much their donation meant to me because words can not describe what an impact it made.

The Husker Power Club has 130 members who have contributed over $2,000 each and 5 members who have contributed over $25,000 each to the strength program. Overall, HPC members have donated nearly 2 million dollars. Other colleges are aware of the success of the Husker Power Club but don't have the support of their athletic director to create a club of their own. I helped Kansas State start a club and shared the paperwork with others, but an athletic director with vision is the key to maintaining a successful booster club for any program.

The bottom line in raising money is it doesn't hurt to ask for help. Every program needs financial help. In the athletic world it seems there is always an item that is needed but never enough money to pay for it. I learned early on in my career that people will donate to improve a facility. If you tell them you need two new platforms with bumper plates and explain how important they will be to your success, you should have no problem raising money from parents or local companies. Where I've run into trouble is trying to raise money for staff. For some reason that is a much more difficult task. It can be done, but it's much harder. A booster club can really make a difference in your strength training facility, but unfortunately not all athletic directors will allow a booster club for strength training.

One of the easiest ways to raise money for us has been to raffle items that were donated by local companies. We sent out one mailing to identify the list of items and ask our boosters to purchase five chances at five dollars each. A second mailing was sent to remind everyone how many days were left with a nice description of the items on the list. You could also add what you plan to do with the money and how it will help your athletes. A third mailing is sent to identify the winners. We averaged six to eight thousand dollars each year for several years until one year I mentioned the raffle to Dan Cook and he said, "Tell your members I'll contribute five dollars for every dollar they contribute up to $60,000. Our members responded by donating $12,000 that year, and he added his $60,000 bringing the total to $72,000. Of course, not every school is going to have a Dan Cook to help, but you can still make an impact without a great amount of additional work. Be sure to check your local raffle regulations.

Equal Support for All Athletes

In 1992, Bill Byrne was hired to replace the legendary Bob Devaney as Nebraska's athletic director. As athletic director at Oregon, Byrne had brought his board of regents into the strength complex when they played Nebraska. He wanted them to see what it would take to be competitive in terms of facilities. I gave them a tour of the facility with no clue that Byrne, who was listening to every word, would one day be my boss. When Byrne was introduced at the student union as the new athletic director at Nebraska, I stood in the back of the room to observe the festivities. I then walked back across campus to my office, and within minutes my secretary called and said, "Bill Byrne and his wife Marilyn are here to see you."

"There's no way," I told her. "I just saw them with Chancellor Spanier across campus a few minutes ago."

She said, "You'd better get down here because it really is Bill Byrne."

I was impressed that Bill and his wife had come to see me first. I was a little concerned, however, that Bill might take away the Husker Power Club and change everything I'd built at Nebraska. I was relieved when Bill said, "I'm excited to be the new athletic director, and I just want to know how I can help. What do you need?"

Tom Osborne had taught me to always be ready with a list of needs in case someone ever asked to help, so I gave Bill a list of three things that had been bothering me and that I wanted to see corrected. He corrected one on the spot, and the other two he entered into his hand-held computer, and within a few weeks they were accomplished also.

Byrne didn't hesitate to demonstrate his great vision, upgrading all sports and their facilities at Nebraska. Few people could follow a legend and be successful, but Bill Byrne clearly showed that he too is a great athletic director. His 10 years were the most successful period in Nebraska history. On December 3, 2002, Bill announced his move to Texas A&M to serve as their athletic director.

In 1993, Bill named me assistant athletic director and asked me to serve on his senior staff of administrators. Bill believed in the concept of an athletic department in which all sports are under one big umbrella. He wanted all Nebraska athletes to be given equal support. He asked me to spread all the services I was providing at the time for football to all the other sports. I told him I would need more staff, and Bill said, "Hire who you need to get the job done."

It took me a while to catch on to Bill's style. For example, when I asked him if I could start a nutritional supplement program, he asked, "How much will it cost?"

"$25,000 a year," I replied.

"Is that just for football?" he asked.

"Yes."

"How much would it be for all of our sports?"

"$40,000," I answered.

Without hesitation, Bill said, "Let's do it for all of them."

Another example of Bill's style occurred a couple of years later. He wanted me to take over the duties of the training table because George Sullivan, the head trainer who had overseen the table for many years, was nearing retirement. I proposed that the strength staff be called the "Performance Team" to include the strength and nutrition staffs, and Bill supported the idea. After a couple of years, Bill asked, "Do you have a female ready to hire full-time from your Performance Team mentoring program?"

I said, "No. We've got Courtney Carter almost ready, but the next person to hire full-time would be Danny Noonan."

Bill said, "Can't we hire both?"

I quickly responded, "Yes, we can."

I was finally catching on to how Bill Byrne wanted things done. In 1996, Courtney Carter became the first full-time female strength coach for Nebraska. She had served as a student strength coach and then as a graduate assistant strength coach as she worked on her master's degree. Courtney is one of the most experienced female strength coaches in the country, handling strength-coaching services for soccer, softball, rifle, and volleyball.

Over time, I made several other changes to better serve the Byrne philosophy. Bill wanted me to make sure all sports had equal access and no one sport was dominant over the others or had special privileges. A policy was established in which all athletes had equal access to the Performance Team facilities. Records and awards were all made equal, regardless of the sport. The Performance Team logo was changed to include a female.

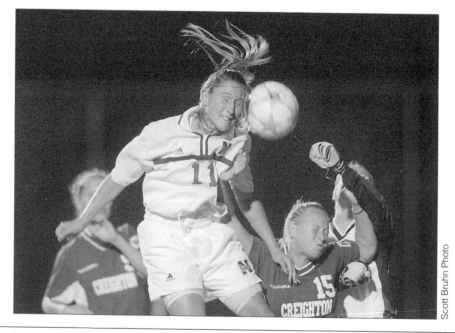

Scott Bruhn Photo

During my time at Nebraska, we took big steps to ensure that Husker Power represented all sports equally.

School records for female sports were displayed in the football stadium. The large words above the mirrors in the strength complex were changed from Nebraska Football to Husker Power to better represent all sports.

Tradition, Teamwork, and Integrity

University of Nebraska Chancellor Harvey Perlman moved quickly to appoint the new Nebraska athletic director 17 days after Bill Byrne resigned to become AD at Texas A&M. Perlman named a 12-member search committee and set a late January date for a hire. Steve Pederson was the forerunner for the position from the start having previously worked at Nebraska as associate athletic director, director of football operations, and recruiting coordinator. The search group didn't even meet before Pederson was hired.

Chancellor Perlman called a meeting of the athletic department to introduce Steve as Nebraska's new AD. Steve earned rave reviews from all corners of the NU athletic department for his enthusiasm and no-nonsense attitude. Although Bill Byrne did a tremendous job for the department, Steve is like a rocket about to take off. There are so many things Nebraska continues to do in its daily routine that are left over from his way of doing business when he was here before. He sets the tone. Under Steve, there would be a new standard for Nebraska employees. People were excited about going to work. Frank Solich said, "Steve has a great understanding of what it's all about in terms of running an athletic department. He'll be the kind of athletic director who moves us all forward." Pederson later told the media, "The only job in the country I would have left Pittsburgh for was Nebraska. This is truly a dream come true for a kid from North Platte. Any team that plans to compete with Nebraska had better bring their A game."

Steve evaluated the staff during his first six months on the job and eliminated 22 positions. He then called a meeting of the remaining 197 athletic department employees and gave each of them a copy of Pat Riley's book *The Warrior Within*. Steve explained how this book detailed the things that he believed are necessary for team building and encouraged the entire staff to read it. He then pointed out that Nebraska is a special place and that as a team we would accomplish great things. He wanted the staff to incorporate three values into everything we did in the future: tradition, teamwork, and integrity. He felt these three words best represent what Nebraska stands for.

Values can be important to team or staff unity. Steve had gathered all the head coaches and asked them what three values best described Nebraska athletics. Then he'd gathered his executive staff and asked them. After much debate these values were selected above the others. They serve as a constant reminder of what we stand for and how we plan to do business. They serve as a guideline in recruiting the type of athletes

Coaches' Support

An example of the kind of support Husker Power receives appears in the entrance of the strength complex. A photo of and quotation from the head coach of each of the 23 sports is included so that any recruit will see his or her sport represented in the facility. Here is a sampling of the quotations:

Gary Pepin, track—"Strength training has played a vital role in the training and performance of the many track and field athletes who have won conference championships and national championships and gone on to compete in the Olympic Games. Thank you Performance Team."

Jay Dirksen, cross country—"Husker Power provides one vital link in the chain of support for all of our student-athletes. The strength, conditioning, and nutrition programs are foundational to their support and ultimate success. We especially appreciate the willingness of Husker Power to adapt these programs to the specific needs of our cross country athletes."

Rhonda Revelle, softball—The Husker strength and conditioning program has had a tremendous impact on our program's success. The strength and power training has helped us reach a new level of explosiveness on the softball field. I am convinced the Husker Power Program is the leader in the field and second to none in collegiate athletics."

John Walker, soccer—"Everybody wants to win on game day, but the few that fulfill this dream do so because of the perseverance, dedication, and "iron-will" shown every day in the weight room."

Pablo Morales, swimming—"Husker Power provides a tremendous strength-building platform upon which to create more powerful swimmers and divers. It has been an integral part of the success of this program."

Dan Kendig, gymnastics—"We not only have the finest strength complex in the country but an excellent staff that is always ready and willing to assist our athletes to maximize their abilities, be it strength, conditioning, flexibility, or nutrition, for optimum performance."

Scott Jacobson, tennis—"The team has benefited every year since the women's tennis team has been taking part in Husker Power. It has helped reduce injuries and add strength, speed, and mobility."

that will feel comfortable and fit into our environment and represent us many years into the future.

In the first few days after my promotion to associate director, Steve asked me to put together a presentation that he could use to generate money for the major construction projects on the horizon. After he saw the presentation, he wrote me a note that said, "Boyd, you have done a great job on our new building project, as I knew you would. It's great to know that I can count on you to deliver at the highest level. . . . You have been the best in your field for four decades; now it's time to become the best at another part of this profession. From what I have seen so far, you are already well on your way to making that happen."

Now that's what I call administrative support. I've had the pleasure of working for Bob Devaney and Tom Osborne and watching their legend stature evolve. Steve Pederson is a perfect fit for Nebraska and will one day be known as the greatest athletic director in history.

Mentoring Program

Many programs have a structure that includes a strength coach, an assistant, a graduate or undergraduate, and a volunteer (see tables 5.1–5.5 for the duties of each). Smaller schools are doing well to have one person assigned to the strength and conditioning program, whereas larger schools have several of each at these levels. Nebraska is constantly being asked to provide strength coaches for other programs. Several years ago, when told Nebraska just didn't have anyone we could afford to lose, the Minnesota Vikings requested permission to send an assistant trainer (Larry Neumann) to Nebraska for a year to learn the Nebraska system. Northern Illinois did the same with Jim Zielinski, who is now a master strength coach.

I have always been faced with the problem of replacing strength coaches. Out of necessity, a mentoring program has evolved. Mike Arthur now heads the mentoring of the student strength coaches.

Job descriptions are provided to identify how the strength coaching structure is set up at many schools. There are many variations to this structure with major schools having several coaches at each level.

An evaluation form is used to determine whether volunteer student strength coaches have potential to be part of the Nebraska Performance Team. Such a form is also used to evaluate student performance each semester. The same kind of form is used to evaluate supervisors (figure 5.1 on page 95).

Athlete Supervision and Motivation

One of the toughest things a strength coach is responsible for is discipline. Athletes expect discipline, but it needs to be consistent for all athletes.

Table 5.1 Director or Head Strength Coach Job Description

I. Reports to

    A. Athletic director

II. Basic Function

    A. Administration of strength and conditioning programs

III. Positions Directly Supervised

    A. Assistant strength coaches

    B. Graduate assistants

    C. Student strength staff and volunteers

IV. Duties and Responsibilities

    A. Develop, distribute, and administer policies and procedures for the staff

    B. Determine the recommended strength and conditioning programs for all sports

    C. Determine lifting technique, reps, sets, and exercises for all sports

    D. Evaluate test scores and oversee body composition plans for all athletes

    E. Evaluate the staff

    F. Oversee budget for program and facilities

    G. Oversee the facility development, use, and inventory of all strength and conditioning equipment

    H. Communicate with coaches as needed for program development

    I. Visit with all recruits, as necessary

    J. Maintain school records and awards; handle press releases

    K. Oversee mentoring of strength coaching staff

    L. Coordinate special events and promotions for strength and conditioning

    M. Attend national strength coaching conventions

Problems develop when someone is getting special treatment or the discipline is different for a starter than for a third-team athlete. Keeping discipline is a matter of telling athletes what is expected of them and explaining the consequences if they don't do it. Bobby Knight, the head basketball coach at Texas Tech University, is known as a strong disciplinarian. He tells his athletes, "Do what needs to be done, when it needs to be done, as well as it can be done, and do it the same way every time."

For over 22 years I punished Nebraska athletes if they missed a workout, class, or practice. They would be required to run stadium steps or do up-and-downs or something similar. In 1991, I developed the Nebraska point system for team discipline. I concluded that punishment is a negative experience for both the athlete and the coach. Many strength coaches are expected to handle discipline for their athletic teams, but it puts them in an awkward position with the athlete. It's harder to motivate athletes to work hard in the weight room if you're also getting them up to run at 6 o'clock

Table 5.2 Assistant Strength Coach Job Description

I. Reports to
    A. Director of athletic performance

II. Basic Function
    A. Assist with the development and administration of strength and conditioning programs

III. Positions Directly Supervised
    A. Graduate assistants
    B. Student strength staff and volunteers

IV. Duties and Responsibilities
    A. Enforce strength and conditioning policies
        1. Enforce daily responsibilities of graduate assistants and student assistants
        2. Enforce compliance of weight room rules, including emergency procedures
    B. Enforce compliance of strength and conditioning principles
        1. Permit only approved exercises to be done in the weight room
        2. Ensure proper exercise techniques
        3. Ensure proper exercise overload
        4. Ensure proper exercise progressions
    C. Program Development and Administration
        1. Assist in developing strength and conditioning programs
            a. winter conditioning
            b. summer conditioning
            c. in-season
            d. bowl preparation
            e. red-shirt programs
            f. incoming freshman programs
            g. take-home summer conditioning manuals
        2. Print lifting program cards for assigned sports
        3. Maintain correct poundage on lifting cards
        4. Keep athlete workout files updated
    D. Testing and Evaluation
        1. Set up for testing
        2. Assist in maintaining database on computer
            a. athlete files
            b. testing records on individual athlete's progress

Table 5.3   Graduate Assistant Job Description

I. Reports to
A. Assistant director
II. Duties and Responsibilities
A. Weight room supervision according to assigned schedule and sports
1. Develop schedule with assistant director
B. Enforce strength and conditioning policies
1. Oversee compliance of daily responsibilities
2. Oversee compliance of weight room rules, including emergency procedures
C. Compliance of strength and conditioning principles
1. Permit only approved exercises to be done in the weight room
2. Ensure proper exercise techniques
3. Ensure proper exercise overload
4. Ensure proper exercise progressions
D. Assist in program development and administration
1. Set up strength program for assigned sports
2. Set up speed and agility program for assigned sports
3. Print lifting program cards for assigned sports
4. Maintain correct poundage on lifting cards
5. Keep individual athlete files updated
E. Assist in testing and evaluation
1. Set up testing for assigned sports
2. Assist in maintaining database on computer
a. assigned player files
b. testing records on individual athletes' progress
c. lifting grades
F. Assist in training students
G. Get certified with the Collegiate Strength and Conditioning Coaches Association
H. Give tours for public relations as needed

in the morning. Most punishment comes in the form of physical activity and, if too demanding, can lead to overtraining. If it isn't hard enough, athletes will soon prefer the punishment to doing the actual workout.

In June of 1991, Coach Osborne asked me to somehow capture the discipline that I maintained in the 1991 winter strength and conditioning program but to ease up on the policy in which an unexcused absence led to dismissal from the team. He wanted a policy that would take into account academic problems and any other violations. I developed a point system based on the national drivers license system. Coach Osborne asked me

Table 5.4 Paid Student Job Description

I. Reports to
   A. Assistant director
II. Duties and Responsibilities
   A. Weight room supervision according to assigned schedule and sports
      1. Develop schedule with assistant director
   B. Work with mentor to enforce strength and conditioning policies
      1. Oversee compliance of daily responsibilities
      2. Oversee compliance of weight room rules including emergency procedures
   C. Work with mentor to enforce strength and conditioning principles
      1. Permit only approved exercises to be done in the weight room
      2. Ensure proper exercise techniques
      3. Ensure proper exercise overload
      4. Ensure proper exercise progressions
   D. Work with mentor to set up strength program for assigned sports
   E. Assist in testing and evaluation
      1. Set up testing for assigned sports

Table 5.5 Volunteer Supervisor Job Description

Objective: To learn and properly demonstrate the following: lifting exercises, warm-up drills, agility drills, speed drills, performance testing; to exhibit knowledge of Performance Team policies and procedures

I. Daily Responsibilities
   A. Be on time for supervision of the strength facility for your assigned times
   B. Wear proper uniform when supervising
   C. Make sure all the weights are in proper place on arrival, while you are on the floor, and before closing
   D. Check for defective equipment and post Do Not Use signs as necessary; report defective equipment to the director
   E. Make sure there's a pen that works at each recording station; if there isn't, replace it
   F. Make sure there's enough wrist straps in the platform area
   G. Make sure the first aid kit is in the supervisor's desk; ensure it's complete
   H. Be sure there's sufficient tape for wrists
   I. Be sure stretching sticks and medicine balls are properly stored
   J. Don't allow football cleats in the weight room
   K. Learn to set up and demonstrate speed and agility drills

(continued)

Table 5.5 *(continued)*

L. Observe and monitor performance and strength testing	
	1. Assist with measuring of vertical jump
	2. Assist with timing of 300-yard shuttle
	3. Watch lines for pro agility and 300-yard shuttle
	4. Assist in office as needed
	5. Learn to answer and operate the phones
M. Learn to set up performance testing equipment	
N. Learn proper active flexibility drills	
O. Learn to perform technique correctly	
	1. Effectively communicate with the lifter to ensure safe proper and effective spotting of a given lift
	2. Make sure bar is evenly loaded and collars are securely fastened
	3. Watch for sliding weights or collars
	4. Try to foresee potential risks of injury, take measures to eliminate, and alert participants of these risks. In the event of an injury, be capable of implementing an emergency medical procedure. (Study emergency procedures.)
	5. Use both hands and proper foot positions when spotting.
	6. Be alert to all changes throughout range-of-motion of a given exercise to assist the lifter when necessary (fatigue, breakdown, or technique).
P. Friday in-season and Wednesday off-season cleaning	
	1. Clean bars with WD40 to remove rust
	2. Put proper amount of chalk in bowls
	3. Lubricate machines
	4. Restock end rolls of tape for wrists
	5. Check fire extinguisher for proper charge

to attend a meeting of his coaches to bring this point system for them to consider. After I presented the concept to the football coaches, Coach Osborne went around the room and asked each coach one at a time if they wanted this point system. He normally didn't make decisions this way, but in this case he wanted complete unity from his staff on this important issue. One at a time they each said yes, and I was asked to implement the point system. The system provided a means for making Nebraska a disciplined team without a lot of punishment, and the result has been team unity. The system is fair to all athletes and includes all support programs, not just the strength and conditioning segment.

How does it work? Athletes are given a point for missing lifting, running, a class, or anything they were asked to attend. Failure to follow instructions also results in a point. Missing a meeting is considered a more serious situation and earns two points, whereas missing a practice is three points.

Husker Power

Evaluator: _____

Evaluation of: _____

For period: _____ **to:** _____

Code
1. Significantly below performance expectations
2. Minimally acceptable performance
3. Meets performance expectations
4. Exceeds performance expectations
5. Clearly exceptional performance

The evaluation process is a method of assessing individual performance. It is an opportunity to bring to light any outstanding contributions or deficiencies among student staff members, and is designed to improve individual job performance, determine appropriate personnel actions, and stimulate individual development.

Communication

    Treats everyone with dignity

    Has the respect of the athletes

    Promotes belief in the Husker Power principles and program

    Has the ability to spot problems and correct mistakes

    Enforces facility rules and policies to athletes

Comments:

	1	2	3	4	5

Responsibility and leadership

    Follows instructions, does not delegate authority, and gets projects done on time

    Behavior consistent with Husker Power policies

    Demonstrates good judgment

    Attendance/promptness

    Quality of work

Comments:

	1	2	3	4	5

Attitude

    Demonstrates loyalty to the program

    Demonstrates trustworthiness and honesty

    Doesn't criticize, complain, or condemn

    Displays good effort and willingness to learn

    Does the recommended lifting program

Comments:

	1	2	3	4	5

Total score

Figure 5.1 Form to evaluate supervisors.

Committing a misdemeanor or academic dishonesty is worth four points, while a felony is worth five points and automatic loss of playing time. See table 5.6 for a chart showing the disciplinary system's standards.

One change in the system occurred after the first year. Originally, when athletes accumulated three points, they would have to go before Coach Osborne to explain the situation. Four points and their parents would be notified. Five points and they would miss the next game. A problem with the original plan was that after accumulating three points, athletes "had" to see Coach Osborne. But Coach Osborne was such a legend that it was actually a privilege for an athlete to get to be in his office. Needless to say, this was not quite the situation we wanted. We didn't want athletes skipping classes, meetings, or practices just to get a few minutes of personal time with Coach Osborne. After the first year, Dr. Jack Stark, the team sports psychologist, created a Unity Council consisting of two players from each position. Now, an accumulation of three points meant athletes had to appear before a council of their peers to explain themselves. This made for a much better deterrent than the "I get to see Coach Osborne" reward.

The Unity Council has also proven to be a great forum for voicing, hearing, and considering athletes' concerns, ranging from whether to

Table 5.6 Nebraska Football Team Policy Standards

Situation	Number of points
Felony conviction	5
Drug policy violation	4
Misdemeanor civil offense	4
Academic dishonesty	4
Unexcused absence from football practice	3
Unexcused absence from team meeting	2
Unexcused absence from lifting session	1
Unexcused absence from conditioning session	1
Unexcused absence from scheduled class	1
Unexcused absence from assigned study hall	1
Unexcused absence from appointment with tutor	1
Failure to follow instructions	1

Each perfect week = 1 point off

Former Nebraska Strength Coaches

The following supervisors helped shape the Husker Power program and have since spread the Nebraska philosophy nationwide. They are listed alphabetically alongside the programs they have represented.

Bill Allerheiligen (Kansas State, Notre Dame, Houston Oilers, Arizona State, Wyoming)

John Archer (Reno, Nevada)

Yon Bakalas (Las Vegas, Nevada)

Dan Barton (Omaha Westside)

Steve Bliss (Miami, Ohio State, North Dakota State)

Aaron Bosket (Oregon State, IUPUI, Indiana)

Mike Butler (Notre Dame)

Kelvin Clark (Vanderbilt, Texas Tech)

Kevin Coleman (Kansas)

Zac Conner (Florida State)

Dr. Larry Crouch (Nebraska Dental College)

Mark Davis (Tennessee State, Vanderbilt)

Lacey Degnan (Montana)

Bill Dorgan (Alabama)

Dave Ellis (Wisconsin)

Steve Fauer (Vanderbilt)

Mike Flynt (Oregon, Texas A&M)

Brian Glover (Colgate)

Tom Halterman (East Chicago High School)

Josh Hingst (Florida State)

David Hofmaier (Idaho State, San Diego Chargers)

Shaun Huls (Reno, Nevada, Hampton)

Joe Hurley (Omaha Gross High School)

John Janecek (Southern Methodist, Tennessee State)

Jon Jost (Holy Cross, Southern Methodist, Florida State)

Brad Junker (Southern Methodist)

Dave Kennedy (Ohio State, Pittsburgh)

Jeff Mangold (Florida, New York Mets, New York Yankees)

(continued)

(continued)

John Maroushek (Ohio State)

Matt Munford (Wyoming)

Jerry Neeman (L.A. Express)

Jared Nessland (North Dakota)

Larry Neumann (Minnesota Vikings)

Zach Nott (Colgate)

Dick Peterson (East Chicago High School)

T.J. Ragan (Colgate, Oregon State)

Dave Redding (Washington State, Missouri, Cleveland Browns, Kansas City Chiefs, Washington Redskins, San Diego Chargers)

Nick Ryan (Illinois)

Jerry Schmidt (Notre Dame, Oklahoma State, Florida, Oklahoma)

Steve Schulz (Stanford)

Kent Stevens (San Francisco Giants)

Donn Swanbom (Southern Methodist, UCLA)

Dr. John Treves (Nebraska Medical Center)

Gary Wade (Detroit Lions, Clemson)

Chris Wieseman (Montana)

Jim Williams (Arkansas, Wyoming, New York Jets, Oklahoma, New York Giants, Philadelphia Eagles)

Tim Wilson (Las Vegas, Nevada, Pittsburgh, Chicago White Sox)

Tom Wilson (Iowa State, California Angels)

Jim Zielinski (Northern Illinois, Oregon State, Illinois)

I extend a sincere thanks to these fine individuals and to the many students who contributed to the success of Husker Power.

allow a player back on the team to which radio station to play in the weight room during workouts. The head coach still has the last word on each issue, but the system allows players a voice. The Unity Council for football has lost some importance in recent years with the development of the Student Advisory Board, which includes athletes from each sport and has representation at NCAA meetings.

The athletic director and head football coach hold the key to success for your strength program. If you have support from both you are on the fast track. If not, you're on a slippery slope.

6

Facilities and Equipment

First impressions are critical when recruiting young athletes, and for most players your program's weight room is a high-profile area. Ideally, you'll want to show off your facilities to your team's future players. This means you need quality equipment in a quality environment. When choosing your facilities and equipment, you need to consider many questions. Will the room have carpet or rubber flooring? Wall treatment or paint? How high should the ceiling be? Can you afford the best strength equipment, dumbbells, plates, and bars that money can buy, or must you go a less expensive route? Here are 10 steps to take on your way to creating the best environment for your players to work in:

1. Determine your needs.
2. Determine actual space available.
3. Determine available equipment inventory.
4. List exercises you want to perform in your new facility.
5. Draw your facility.
6. Determine new equipment to add.
7. Determine your budget.
8. Order your equipment.
9. Teach proper use of new equipment.
10. Maintain all equipment properly.

Step 1: Determine Your Needs

Not everyone can afford the top-of-the-line brand of equipment. Many companies sell low-quality products. These companies tend to come and go, but their low-quality products continue to show up in our high schools. We don't recommend purchasing low-quality products. In the long run, you get what you pay for in terms of durability and dependability. Look for reasonably priced but safe and effective equipment.

Give serious consideration to what level of quality you want in your facility. Of course, you want a facility that makes you proud to show it to people, but it's possible to overdo the luxury for athletes in an attempt to impress them. Too much luxury or gaudiness in a weight room can be seen as a negative to those who need to use the facility daily. There's a fine line between a show place and a room that motivates athletes to work harder to improve. A facility that is well lighted, colorful, and motivating to the people using it will produce the best results.

In addition to aesthetics, you'll want to determine your needs in terms of what your lifting program calls for. If you train athletes and not just students, you'll want to include explosive training that requires lifting platforms and bumper plates. The students might not use them, but your athletes will benefit from them a great deal. Platforms with your school logo on them work wonders in terms of aesthetics and motivation. If your facility includes physical education classes, you'll want to consider a circuit-training area and an aerobic area for fitness. You'll need to know class size and design a program to handle that number of students. If your facility will be open to the public, you'll need more fitness machines and you might want to consider a secured area for your free-weight equipment.

Supervision Area

An office with windows that provides a clear view of the room is best. Some facilities have room for only a desk or counter. Better security is needed for important papers, the stereo, and other valuables. A counseling room adjacent to the office is great because it provides a private setting for you to talk to your athletes. The counseling room could also serve as a mini-library with resource materials relating to strength, conditioning, and nutrition.

Supervision Area Checklist

Phone with emergency numbers

Desk and chair

Music source (secured)

Light switches (except for emergency and security lights)

Filing system

Computer

Warm-Up Area

Nebraska uses two warm-up exercises in the weight room, which work very well. The first exercise involves gliding under a hurdle for two sets of 10 reps. You'll want to include 8 to 10 hurdles if space allows so that several athletes can do the hurdle stretch together. The hurdle should not have a cross-bar that prevents gliding underneath it. The second warm-up exercise is the squat snatch, for which you'll need two or three light bars. Use a light weight for the squat snatch and perform two warm-up sets of five reps. Look for illustrations of the squat snatch in the exercise section.

Warm-Up Area Checklist

Hurdles

Light Olympic warm-up bars (25-pound, 45-pound, and 75-pound bars)

Stretching sticks

Coach Epley's tip: Allen High School in Allen, Texas, uses light bars in their 24 power racks to simulate a hurdle to glide under for the hurdle warm-up. They use the same light bars and stay inside the power racks to perform the squat snatch warm-up.

Explosive Training Area

When possible, keep this area away from the traffic flow to avoid some-one walking too close to an athlete doing explosive lifts. At Nebraska, we normally recommend 8-foot-by-8-foot platforms, but after training at USC for the Rose Bowl we discovered their 8-foot-by-6-foot platforms space worked fine for power cleans. The 8-foot-by-10-foot platforms we recommend have half-racks on them but allow room for power cleans from the floor. Olympic bars are needed on the platform as well as bumper plates to protect the floor. Platforms allow for the best and safest plan for explosive lifting. Powerlift platforms can be purchased in sizes of 8-foot width by 4-foot, 8-foot, 10-foot, or 12-foot length.

A big part of any explosive area are the bumper plates used on the lifting platforms. Nebraska asked Usesaka of Japan to make bumper plates in pounds rather than kilos for exercises in which the bar touches the ground. Converting kilos to pounds can be time consuming, and for years our athletes and coaches were confused about how much weight was on the bar. With pound plates instead of the metric plates, we always know exactly how much we're lifting.

Another important part of explosive lifting is a safe rack to train on. For lifts done overhead, such as the push press or push jerk, you need a power rack so that these explosive exercises are safe. Most equipment

One year we were allowed to use the Phoenix College wrestling room for our lifting at the Fiesta Bowl. Normally, visiting teams are not allowed this luxury. The athletic director at Phoenix College, former wrestling coach Ron Easton, was extremely protective of this space. But because I had graduated from Phoenix College, Coach Easton agreed to let our players train in his wrestling room. The wrestling mats were removed, which left a basketball-type wood floor. We put a light rubber mat over the floor to protect it from scuffing, but it was not thick enough to prevent damage from dropping weights. So I instructed our players not to drop the Olympic bar as they came in after practice and lifted. Everyone got the message but Kenny Walker, who is deaf and didn't hear the warnings. He was lifting several hundred pounds and dropping them on the thin mat. By the time I got over to stop him, he had destroyed a large enough area that we had to replace the entire wood floor. It's pretty funny to think about now, but at the time Coach Easton wasn't impressed.

companies now offer power racks in three basic styles with a variety of options (figure 6.1).

The three power-rack choices include the four-post rack, which has been available for many years and provides the most stability. The power rack features four large posts, dual-grip chin-up bar, safety spot bars, and weight storage. This rack provides a large enclosed work area for the athlete where safety may be the main issue.

The four-post multi-rack is a shorter version of the power rack that was designed and tested at Nebraska. The multi-rack has four shorter posts and also works well with bench or incline. This rack provides many of the same features as the power rack with a more open design. Also the bar can easily be taken over the front post to work outside the rack. The rear post can be ordered taller for adding a chin-up bar as well.

The two-post half-rack, also developed at Nebraska, is the most economical and efficient rack. The half-rack with a bench is an especially good buy. All the same lifts can be performed here with the exception of a front military press due to the lack of the front post. Many like the open design, which takes up less space in the weight room.

The half-rack is also shown with technique trays for hang cleans. The half-rack with technique trays is best for hang cleans on a wood platform insert. These trays are solid supports for bumper plates and adjustable to various heights. The half-rack post can also be ordered taller for adding a chin-up bar.

All three kinds of power rack provide a variety of exercises and options, such as wooden platform inserts. Go to power-lift.com for more details and features.

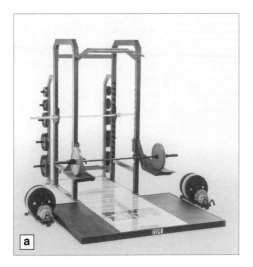
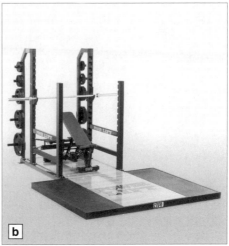
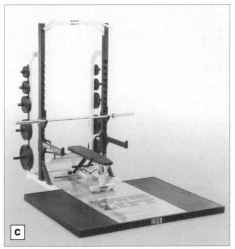
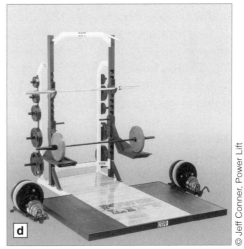

© Jeff Conner, Power Lift

Figure 6.1 *(a)* Power rack, *(b)* multi-rack, *(c)* half-rack, and *(d)* half-rack with technique trays.

Explosive Training Area Checklist

Platforms

Olympic bars

Locks for Olympic bars

Bumper plates (45 and 25 pounds)

Plates (2.5, 5, and 10 pounds)

Plate racks

Hammer jammers

Rubber-coated plates or bumpers for jammers (25 and 45 pounds)

Plates for jammers (2.5, 5, and 10 pounds)

Power rack, multi-rack, or half-rack

Coach Epley's tip: To save space and cost, look closely at the half-rack with technique trays and a wooden platform insert. Some schools combine the explosive area exercises with the slow-movement area exercises and do both on the same racks. Choose your program, then arrange your facility to allow athletes to work under close supervision.

Slow-Movement Area

A slow-movement area has three basic formats to choose from: single station, multiexercise station, and circuit training. Nebraska uses a combination of the three.

The single-station concept calls for an individual station for each exercise. For example, a station for the bench press, another station for the incline press, another for the shoulder press, and so on.

The multiexercise station format calls for multiple exercises to be done at one station. The multiexercise station provides versatility, with squats and cleans being done at the same station as bench or shoulder presses. The multiexercise station concept allows the room to handle many students at once, but please provide supervision. A room full of multiexercise stations can be pretty impressive—just look at Arizona State's 28 multiexercise stations in one room (see page 124). Everyone can do squats or cleans at once. Give some thought to what your major exercises are and how many stations you can supervise. The technical lifts, such as the hang clean and squat, require close supervision.

Rather than positioning the racks all along one wall, you might consider an arrangement with two rows that allows better supervision by placing the tall part of the rack to the outside and the low part to the inside. This creates an alley effect, so the supervisor can better see all lifts done in both rows at the same time. If you go this route, be sure to leave at least five feet between rows.

The multiexercise station concept was developed by Donn Swanbom at UCLA in 1973. Donn had been an assistant strength coach at Nebraska. He created a system using power racks to train a large number of athletes in a small space.

Nebraska always had a larger area to work with than most schools had, so we never used the true multiexercise station system. We prefer specialization over versatility. We like doing bench presses in racks designed for the bench press and squats in racks designed for squats. We assign supervisors based on the lift they are trained to supervise. For example, we do squat and bench (slow movements) one day and clean and jammer (explosive movements) the next day in different areas of the weight room.

The third approach is circuit training, in which the exerciser rotates from station to station until the circuit is completed. The circuit can consist of a machine or free weights or a combination of the two.

Choose the program you want to use before arranging your circuit equipment. Determine how many students you have and how much time they'll need to complete the circuit. This information is necessary to determine how many stations to include in the circuit, how many sets can be done, and how much rest between stations is required. To handle many students at once in a fitness circuit, it's best to set up several stations of exercises that aren't overly demanding. Although only 8 to 10 stations are required for a balanced program, some fitness circuits have 15 or more stations to accommodate the number of students in a class. For example, if there are 30 students in a class, the circuit might need to consist of 15 stations, with pairs of students working together at each station as they move through the circuit. If they each did two sets at each of the 15 stations, the program would take about 30 minutes.

Slow-Movement Area Checklist

Adjustable bench

Work benches

Dumbbells

Dumbbell rack

Specialty bars, plates, and plate racks

High pulley

Low pulley

Hammer leverage machines

Standing leg curl

8 to 15 circuit stations

Hammer push–pull circuit

Coach Epley's tip: When possible, place the tall objects to the outside of your facility to prevent obstruction of the supervisor's view. This creates an alley from which the supervisor can see all exercises at once. When several half-racks are placed back to back with the tall portion to the inside, it's impossible for one person to supervise all the athletes as they perform their major lifts.

Aerobic Area

This area should be well ventilated with good natural light. TVs and music are expected frills in this area.

Aerobic Area Checklist

TV

Treadmills

Bikes

Cross-trainers

Rowers

Coach Epley's tip: Look for cross-trainers that are portable and don't need electrical power. Most aerobic equipment requires electrical cords, which can be safety hazards.

Agility Area

The agility area needs to be in an area free of obstacles. Ohio State and Texas Tech have a fieldhouse adjacent to their weight room, whereas Texas, Texas A&M, and others have turf for agility drills or pulling sleds right inside their weight rooms. A good safe surface is difficult to find, so many programs are not able to do agility drills properly.

Agility Area Checklist

Four lines painted 5 yards apart

6 to 8 cones 6 to 12 inches high

Nutrition Area

Years ago, before nutritional supplements were available, athletes ate more food to add calories. Rod Horn, a defensive lineman at Nebraska, drank a gallon of milk and ate a loaf of bread dipped in a bowl of gravy along with each meal. His 5,000 to 6,000 calories per meal made national news.

Nutritional supplements have become more important and popular in recent years, and an area to keep them should be incorporated into any new facility. Distributing supplements can be a problem because some athletes will want them when they don't need them, and others won't want them when they would benefit from them. Let's run through a quick overview on how we view nutrition at Nebraska. We place concerns about nutrition into three categories: hydration, recovery, and prescription.

All athletes need to be hydrated during workouts. Jet sprays can mix drinks well for hydration, but the jet spray machines need to be cleaned and filled regularly, which requires more manpower than most programs have. At Nebraska, we use a system in which the fluid comes in a bag. It's called the "bag-in-the-box" system and allows for quick access.

Recovery after workouts is the second area of nutrition. Some athletes are trying to lose weight and don't need excess calories. Supplements contain extra calories and should be limited for these athletes. Distribution is also a problem for recovery supplements. In a small facility, a student manager could distribute the cans or bars to athletes who need them. Some current research indicates it might be a good idea to also give supplements before the workout.

The third area involves supplements recommended or prescribed by coaches that an athlete would take home to gain or lose weight. Be sure to keep accurate records of any recommendations you make to an athlete.

Nutrition Area Checklist

Water coolers

Supplement dispensers

Trash containers

Coach Epley's tip: Make sure everyone drinks plenty of water or Gatorade each day. Only give recovery supplements to students who are trying to gain weight; establish a system in which only the intended students have access to their daily supply.

Storage and Receiving Room and Tool Room

Determine the width of the doorway through which equipment will be brought into the facility. A 36-inch doorway won't work as well as a 40-inch doorway. In any case, a double-door or garage door, if available, is probably best for getting equipment in and out of your facility. If that's not possible, a double-wide doorway with a removable post usually works fine. Texas has a great setup for receiving equipment. They have a drive leading up to a receiving room adjacent to the weight room with a garage door on the outside and a double-door that enters the weight room. This provides an opportunity to put equipment together or test it before it goes on the floor of the facility. This area could also serve as a tool room for repairs.

At Nebraska, we have an extensive supply of tools, including a welder, air compressor, and an assortment of saws and drills. Many schools might not have a person on hand like our Randy Gobel, who oversees equipment and facility repairs and uses a wide variety of tools, but every tool room should be stocked with at least the basic tools needed to put together and take apart equipment.

Tool Room Checklist

Hammer, pliers, screwdrivers

Allen wrench, crescent wrench

Carpet knife, heavy-duty stapler

Duct tape, scotch tape, masking tape

Drill and drill bits

Lubricant spray and spray paints to match equipment

Staff Locker Room

Plan ahead! Many of the best facilities don't have a staff locker room for supervisors to change and shower. This is an area that's far from mandatory, but it will be missed if not included at your facility.

Staff Locker Room Checklist

Lockers (built in) that lock

Towels

Restroom with sink and mirror

Laundry system

Seats

Trash can

Scale

Door that locks

Lunch Room

Larger facilities might require a lunch room (sometimes called a break room). Anticipate your needs and how this room would be used by your athletes and staff.

Lunch Room Checklist

Sink

Refrigerator

Table and chairs

Television

Microwave

Glassware

Cabinets

Restroom for Athletes

Believe it or not, restrooms are sometimes forgotten. You don't need anything fancy, but every facility should include a men's room and women's room.

Restroom Checklist

Unisex restroom with one toilet, sink, and mirror

Door that locks

Step 2: Determine
Actual Space Available

Whether you're dealing with an existing facility or a blueprint of a new facility, identify any permanent fixtures that can't be altered, such as doors, pipes, windows, and mirrors. A light switch, for example, can prevent placing a mirror where you want. Most light switches are four feet from the ground, whereas electrical outlets should be one foot off the ground. Mirrors should be placed 34 inches above the floor to avoid being broken by dumbbells being placed in the dumbbell rack. As for pipes or protrusions on the wall, adjust to anything you can't move, such as air conditioning duct work.

A 10- to 12-foot minimum ceiling height is recommended for school lifting areas. The higher the ceiling, the more impressive your facility will be. Some facilities have 40-foot ceilings. Be sure to factor in heating costs when deciding how high to make your ceilings.

It might be a hassle, but you should know exactly where everything will be placed in your new facility before ordering anything. Don't make the too-common error of ordering equipment that won't fit well into the allotted space. Follow each step in this chapter to avoid problems with planning your facility.

Coach Epley's tip: Avoid putting equipment in front of a walk lane that leads to a fire exit.

Step 3: Determine
Available Equipment Inventory

Make a list of the condition of your existing equipment and determine what should be repaired, what needs new upholstery, and what needs to be replaced. With a little work, some equipment can be spruced up and look like new again. Preacher curl pads can be replaced. Weights can be painted. Some schools paint their weights different colors to help keep them in a certain area. Outdated equipment that can't be repaired should be replaced.

Coach Epley's tip: You might be able to generate some income for new equipment by selling the equipment you want to replace. If you choose to try this, be sure to go through the proper channels. More than one strength coach has lost his job for selling school property.

Step 4: List Exercises You Want to Perform in Your New Facility

Match the equipment list from step three to a list of exercises you want to do in your program. Circle or mark exercises for which you don't have the proper equipment so you know what you need to order. If you're planning on explosive lifting and you don't have a lifting platform with bumper plates, you'll need to add these to your purchase list.

Step 5: Draw Your Facility

Identify all permanent fixtures, and then, using a quarter-inch to one-foot scale, create drawings that include all the equipment you intend to place in the facility. Allow enough space to walk around equipment and get in and out of it safely. Include plenty of space for spotters to do their job. Don't place equipment too close to walls, pillars, or mirrors. If athletes' bodies will extend out from equipment during use, be sure to allow space for this. Also allow enough space for traffic flow through the facility to exits.

Place sit-up boards and stretching mats well out of the way of lifting areas. It's imperative that the matted areas are far enough away from the overhead lifting areas to avoid any hazards that could result from weights falling or being dropped.

Assess your program needs and arrange your equipment accordingly. You might want to group the major lifting stations together in different areas of the room from the stations that don't require as much supervision. The weight room arrangement really depends on personal preference, but make sure that traffic flow in and out of the facility doesn't interfere with the lifting or spotting of the athletes' lifting. Nebraska has a carpeted circuit area, a wooden platform area for squats and cleans, and a rubber floor area for supplemental machines.

Coach Epley's tip: Creating a drawing is a little extra work but allows you to determine where everything goes before you order anything new. It's a lot easier to move equipment on a piece of paper than it is in real life.

Since coaches won't necessarily have the detailed computer drawing available to design their facility, I have included an identical drawing with rectangular boxes in place of the particular pieces of equipment (see figure 6.2). This should allow any coach to determine spaces needed in their facility.

Jefferson High School had a make-over to include explosive lifting, a push–pull circuit and a metabolic circuit (figure 6.3). These changes allowed their facility to provide for all the recommended programs in this book.

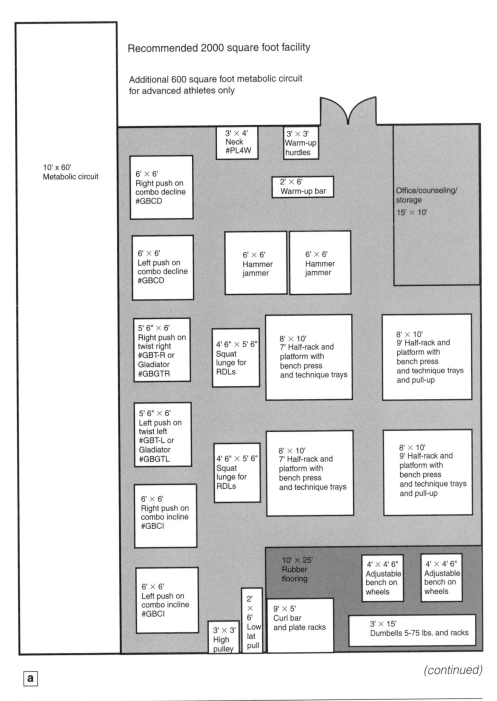

Recommended 2000 square foot facility

Additional 600 square foot metabolic circuit
for advanced athletes only

10' x 60'
Metabolic circuit

3' × 4'
Neck
#PL4W

3' × 3'
Warm-up
hurdles

6' × 6'
Right push on
combo decline
#GBCD

2' × 6'
Warm-up bar

Office/counseling/
storage
15' × 10'

6' × 6'
Left push on
combo decline
#GBCD

6' × 6'
Hammer
jammer

6' × 6'
Hammer
jammer

5' 6" × 6'
Right push on
twist right
#GBT-R or
Gladiator
#GBGTR

4' 6" × 5' 6"
Squat
lunge for
RDLs

8' × 10'
7' Half-rack and
platform with
bench press
and technique trays

8' × 10'
9' Half-rack and
platform with
bench press
and technique trays
and pull-up

5' 6" × 6'
Left push on
twist left
#GBT-L or
Gladiator
#GBGTL

4' 6" × 5' 6"
Squat
lunge for
RDLs

8' × 10'
7' Half-rack and
platform with
bench press
and technique trays

8' × 10'
9' Half-rack and
platform with
bench press
and technique trays
and pull-up

6' × 6'
Right push on
combo incline
#GBCI

10' × 25'
Rubber
flooring

4' × 4' 6"
Adjustable
bench on
wheels

4' × 4' 6"
Adjustable
bench on
wheels

6' × 6'
Left push on
combo incline
#GBCI

2'
×
6'
Low
lat
pull

9' × 5'
Curl bar
and plate racks

3' × 15'
Dumbells 5-75 lbs. and racks

3' × 3'
High
pulley

a

(continued)

Figure 6.2 Recommended facility *(a)* with equipment spaces identified as rectangular boxes and *(b)* with equipment drawings.

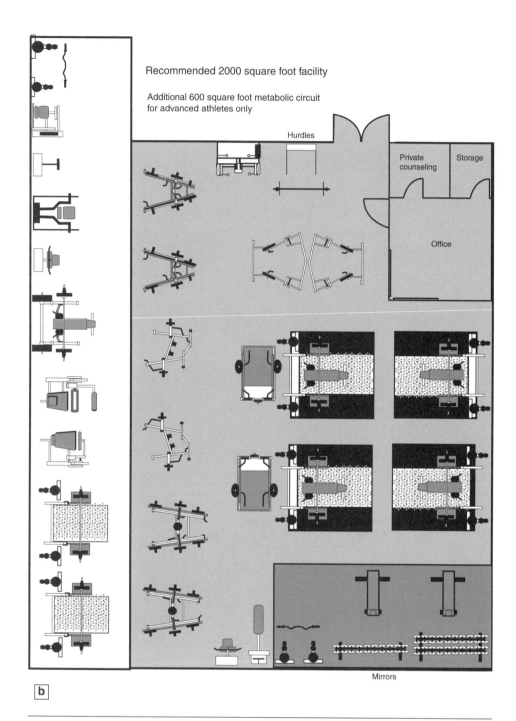

Recommended 2000 square foot facility

Additional 600 square foot metabolic circuit for advanced athletes only

Hurdles

Private counseling

Storage

Office

Mirrors

b

Figure 6.2 *(continued)*

112

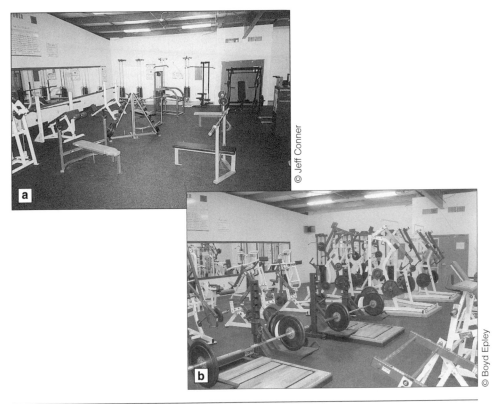

© Jeff Conner

© Boyd Epley

Figure 6.3   *(a)* Before and *(b)* after photos of Jefferson High School.

Step 6: Determine
New Equipment to Add

Determine how the items you need will be purchased. Don't forget to include shipping costs, and allow at least eight weeks for delivery. Ask the manufacturer about crating costs or other hidden costs in getting the equipment to your facility properly set up and in working order. Ask if the equipment needs to be bolted down or put together before use. Include all foreseeable costs in your budget.

You might have to prioritize your list of needs and wants in order of importance and get approval from your athletic trainer or another supervisor. Remember that there's a difference between what you want for your program and what you actually need. The athletic director will appreciate accurate figures. The more organized you are in your submitted request, the better chance you have of getting everything approved.

When selecting equipment, be sure the equipment you're choosing does what you want it to do. Look at frame construction—can it stand the rigor of continuous use by athletes? Are joints welded and ground smooth? Is the equipment simple to use and safe? Will the company you're buying from be around in five years when you need new parts, cables, or upholstery? Does the equipment adjust to the size of your athletes? Do the machines have heavy enough weight stacks?

Take extra time in selecting the basic equipment you'll use every day so that you're not surprised with what you receive. There are many kinds of bars, dumbbells, and bumper plates out there, so do the necessary research before you buy.

- *Bars.* Three types of bars are recommended: (1) Usesaka bars for use on platforms; (2) powerlift bars for bench press, squat racks, and general exercises; and (3) 15-pound aluminum bars for warm-up exercises. The platform bars should be of the highest quality, with needle bearings that allow for a quick turn under the bar when lifting and a solid end-piece securing the sleeve.
- *Dumbbells.* No piece of equipment takes more of a beating than dumbbells. Think durability. Also, do you want dumbbells that increase in 2-1/2-pound or 5-pound increments? Do you want knurling on the handle or not? Do you want solid or plate dumbbells? Also order heavy duty racks to hold the dumbbells.
- *Bumper plates.* Select plates completely covered in rubber. They last longer than the iron plates surrounded by a rubber strip. Consider whether you want your plates in pounds or kilograms. Usesaka is the company that provides metric bumper plates for the Olympic Games. In 2002, they teamed with Power Lift to produce a 20-inch all-rubber bumper in pounds. Standard bumper plates used to be 18 inches, but because athletes are getting bigger, plates are larger so that athletes don't have to bend as far to lift them off the ground, thus improving leverage. Colorado was the first university to use these new bumper plates.

Coach Epley's tip: Equipment is purchased or donated for many reasons. You should evaluate the equipment in your facility at least once a year, assessing what you need and don't need. If the equipment is not being used in your program, why let it take up valuable space in the weight room?

A high school could do a balanced program in the recommended weight room without metabolic equipment (table 6.1). The metabolic equipment is listed separately (table 6.2). All schools will have a weight room but not all will have the luxury of space for a metabolic circuit.

Table 6.1 Recommended Equipment List

Model #	Items from Life Fitness or Hammer	Weight	Comments	Number
GBJ	Jammer		Specify color of unit and lever arms	2
	Plates for Jammer	45 lb	Coated would be quieter than cast iron	12
		25 lb	Local cast-iron plates	4
		10 lb	Local cast-iron plates	4
		5 lb	Local cast-iron plates	8
H-hornassy	Additional weight horns for Jammer			4
H-horn-hrdwe-asy	Hardware for attaching weight horns			4
GBSL	Squat lunge machine for RDLs		Specify color	2
	Plates for squat lunge machine	45 lb	Local cast-iron plates	12
		25 lb	Local cast-iron plates	4
		10 lb	Local cast-iron plates	4
FWDR1	Single dumbbell rack		Specify color	1
FWDR2	Two-tier dumbbell rack		Specify color	1
	Dumbbells	5-25 lb	Iron Grip local brand	1
	Dumbbells	30-50 lb	Iron Grip local brand	1
	Dumbbells	55-75 lb	Iron Grip local brand	1
	Push–pull circuit			
GBCI	Combo incline for push–pull circuit		Specify color	2
GBT-R	Twist right for push–pull circuit		Specify color	1
GBT-L	Twist left for push–pull circuit		Specify color	1
GBCD	Combo decline for push–pull circuit		Specify color	2
	Plates for push–pull circuit	45 lb	Local cast-iron plates	24
		25 lb	Local cast-iron plates	12
		10 lb	Local cast-iron plates	12
H-hornassy	Additional weight horns for push–pull circuit			24

(continued)

Table 6.1 *(continued)*

Model #	Items from Life Fitness or Hammer	Weight	Comments	Number
H-horn-hrdwe-asy	Hardware for attaching weight horns			4
SU45	Hi-lat pull-down station with seat			1
SU50	Low-lat pull with seat			1
	Shipping from Life Fitness			

Model #	Items from Power Lift	Weight	Comments	Number
	Platforms			
OP88I	8 in. × 8 in. wood platform tops for clean platforms			4
HFR	7-in. half-racks			2
HFR-9	9-in. half-racks come with pull-up			2
TT	Technique scoops		Pairs	4
CSBC-45	Bumper plates for platform lifts	45 lb	Usesaka from Power Lift	24
CSBC-25	Bumper plates for platform lifts	25 lb	Usesaka from Power Lift	8
	Plates for platform lifts	10 lb	Local cast-iron plates	8
		5 lb	Local cast-iron plates	16
		2.5 lb	Local cast-iron plates	8
PBEN	Lever action bench			4
PL4W	Four-way neck with rubber feet			1
	Additional weight horns for neck			3
	Cast-iron plates for neck	45 lb	Local cast-iron plates	1
		25 lb	Local cast-iron plates	1
		10 lb	Local cast-iron plates	2
PDBB	Adjustable benches		With wheels	2
	EZ-curl bar		Local	1
	Plates for EZ-curl bar	45 lb	Local cast-iron plates	2
		25 lb	Local cast-iron plates	2
		10 lb	Local cast-iron plates	2
		5 lb	Local cast-iron plates	4
		2.5 lb	Local cast-iron plates	2

(continued)

Model #	Items from Power Lift	Weight	Comments	Number
FWDWT	Plate racks for E-Z curl bar			2
AL 15	Warm-up bar from solid bar	15 lb	Aluminum	1
CSBC-25	Bumper plates for warm-up bar	25 lb	Usesaka from Power Lift	2
	Shipping from Power Lift			
Model #	Additional items	Weight	Comments	Number
	Warm-up hurdle		Local	6
UG-158 TW	Olympic bar from Usesaka		For platform lifts	4
	Locks for platforms and jammers from Husker Power		Two for warm-up and two for curl bar	16
	Sound system			
	Supplements and dispenser			
	Storage racks for store room			
	Mirrors for dumbbell area		4 ft × 8 ft	
	Record board			
	Tools			
	Desk and chair			
	Water fountain			
	Computer			
	Scale			1
	Skinfold calipers			
	Carpet or rubber flooring			

Table 6.2 Recommended Metabolic Equipment List

Model #	Metabolic circuit	Weight	Comments	Number
CC8152	Pro Time circuit interval timer			1
HFR	Warm-up and squat in half-racks		Need technique scoops for safety level	2

(continued)

Table 6.2 *(continued)*

Model #	Metabolic circuit	Weight	Comments	Number
OP88I	8 in. × 8 in. wood platform tops			2
	Plates for squat	45 lb	Local cast-iron plates	12
		25 lb	Local cast-iron plates	4
		10 lb	Local cast-iron plates	4
		5 lb	Local cast-iron plates	8
		2.5 lb	Local cast-iron plates	4
PLPB	Powerlift bar for squat	45 lb		2
	Locks for squat from Husker Power			4
S140	Leg curl			1
S120	Leg extension			1
	Bench press in 7-ft half-rack			1
PBEN	Lever action bench			1
PLPB	Powerlift bar for bench press	45 lb		1
	Plates for bench press	45 lb	Local cast-iron plates	6
		25 lb	Local cast-iron plates	2
		10 lb	Local cast-iron plates	2
		5 lb	Local cast-iron plates	4
		2.5 lb	Local cast iron plates	2
	Locks for bench from Husker Power			2
SU45	High pulley with seat			1
SU25	Shoulder press machine			1
FSLP	Standing low lat pull		No seat	1
FSHP	High pulley without seat for triceps extension			1
	Curl bar		Local	1
FWDWT	Curl-bar plate racks			2
	Curl-bar plates	45 lb	Local cast-iron plates	2
		25 lb	Local cast-iron plates	2
		10 lb	Local cast-iron plates	2
		5 lb	Local cast-iron plates	4
		2.5 lb	Local cast-iron plates	2

Step 7: Determine Your Budget

When pricing equipment before purchasing, be sure to get current quotes from equipment companies. Prices go up from time to time, and if you're on a tight budget an increase can put you over budget. Most pieces of equipment are direct purchases with funds raised through a booster club, private donations, and fund-raising projects, but some companies allow equipment to be leased over several years.

After determining your budget, you can go back and make final adjustments to your facility design. Add in the new equipment that your budget allows with the existing equipment and arrange equipment based on traffic flow, safety, and supervision that will be required. The supervision requirements should be considered early on in the facility design.

Coach Epley's tip: When planning your budget, don't forget to add in the cost of repairing the old equipment.

Step 8: Order Your Equipment

Order early, allowing at least eight weeks for delivery time and installation. I recommend doing the ordering yourself so that you're confident everything has been ordered precisely to your specifications. That way, if something doesn't arrive, or if the wrong piece of equipment comes in place of one you ordered, you know a mistake has been made on the supplier's part, and you can take the steps to correct the error as quickly as possible.

Coach Epley's tip: Have a copy of your facility drawing ready when the equipment arrives and have a spot waiting for the equipment so everyone knows where to put it. This will save a lot of time and energy.

Step 9: Teach Proper Use of New Equipment

Teach good technique and safety, especially in the lifting area. Show athletes how to use all new equipment. The natural tendency for people is to want to see what the "new toy" can do. The first few minutes that the new equipment is on the floor of the weight room is the best time to teach athletes how to use it. If instructions are provided, post them in a place where everyone can see them. Always make sure there's enough supervision in the weight room. Younger and less experienced athletes require more supervision than older or more experienced athletes. For junior high strength and conditioning facilities, there should be at least one supervisor for every 10 students. For high school facilities, there should be one supervisor for every 15 students. Facilities that serve athletes older than high school age should have at least one supervisor for every 20 students. Ideally, these numbers result in one strength and conditioning coach per three training stations or each 1,000 square feet of area for junior high weight rooms; one per five training stations or 1,500 square feet for high school weight rooms; and one per six to seven training stations or 2,000 square feet of area for college weight rooms.

Athletes engaged in circuit training with resistance machines don't require as much supervision as athletes performing explosive lifts or technical lifts, such as the squat. The supervisor station should have a clear view of the lifting room. Keep a stocked first aid box, and know where it is at all times. Keep the air temperature of the facility constant between 72 and 78 degrees. Post weight room rules, regulation policies, safety procedures, and emergency phone numbers near the entrance or by the supervisors' station in clear view.

There are several basic steps that all strength coaches should take to make their weight rooms safe for their athletes:

- Obtain preparticipation medical clearance for all athletes prior to the season.
- Ensure that all supervisors have proper credentials and training.
- Maintain a good coach-to-athlete ratio.
- Put athletes through orientation.
- Use proper equipment purchasing and spacing.
- Perform daily maintenance.

Let your athletes know what they should do if an injury occurs. In the event of an accident, be ready to handle the situation as quickly and efficiently as possible. Your weight room should have an easily accessible emergency plan approved by your athletic director.

Whenever new athletes come into the weight room, there should be a formal orientation to provide them with an overview of safety rules and behavior expectations (see table 6.3).

Coach Epley's tip: Make sure the stereo system is not played so loud that spotters and lifters can't hear each other clearly. Some athletes like the music so loud they can "feel it," but their safety is more important.

It's hard to imagine a weight room without a radio, but Nebraska went three years without one. Freshman Bob Martin, who later became an All-American defensive end, donated Nebraska's first weight room radio in December 1972. Thanks to a donation from Dan Cook, a booster from Dallas, the current strength complex has three different types of speakers in a sophisticated sound system, including speakers for music, voice, and video. Music can be motivating in a lifting facility but can also get out of control. There are many ways to control what type of music is played. At one time Nebraska had "Country Thursday," where country music was played all day. The music is now controlled by the Student Athlete Advisory Board, which represents all Nebraska athletes. They determine what station will be selected. If an athlete doesn't like the music, they can discuss it with their advisory board representative.

Step 10: Maintain All Equipment Properly

Keep a record of equipment use and maintenance in case there's an injury and you need to provide information. Document anything unusual and every change or adaptation to the equipment. Create a checklist to use daily, weekly, monthly, and annually.

> *Daily*—when you arrive each day and before you leave, walk the floor to make sure everything is working properly and is put back where it belongs.
>
> *Weekly*—clean and disinfect benches.
>
> *Monthly*—lubricate bars and tighten bolts on machines.
>
> *Annually*—replace worn upholstery; replace equipment that is not used.

Although high school coaches aren't manufacturing or selling strength equipment, they can still be named as codefendants in product liability suits. Two key factors are examined in the event of an injury and lawsuit: (1) whether the equipment has been changed from the condition in which it was originally sold and (2) whether the equipment was being used as intended by the manufacturer.

To protect yourself from a lawsuit, do the following:

- Use the equipment only for the purpose intended by the manufacturer.

- Be certain equipment meets existing professional standards. Don't buy unsafe equipment.
- Buy only from reputable manufacturers. If you're not sure who to buy from, ask colleagues for recommendations.
- Apply all warning labels that accompany a new equipment purchase.
- Continually inspect equipment for damage and wear that may place an athlete at risk.
- Don't allow unsupervised athletes to use equipment.
- Use proper technique when using the equipment.
- Machines with electric cords should be kept as close to walls as possible. If an athlete has to step over or near a cord, it should be covered and secured.

Coach Epley's tip: If you modify the equipment in any way, even something as simple as changing a cable, write it down and include the date. If anyone is ever injured, the court will appreciate your records on maintenance of the equipment.

Table 6.3   Weight Room Rules

Failure to follow any of these rules could result in loss of weight room privileges.

1. Before participation, athletes must have a medical check-up.

2. Before participation, all athletes must undergo an orientation on common risks involved in strength training, on the proper execution of exercises, and on the possible consequences if proper technique is not employed.

3. Athletes are to receive a workout program card from the strength coach, follow it, and record workout contents.

4. If an athlete has an injury that in any way inhibits a portion of the workout, the coach should provide the athlete with a modified program outlining which movements are to be avoided and which might be substituted.

5. Athletes are required to use collars once there's more than one plate on the end of the bar.

6. Athletes move weights from the racks to the bar only. They never set plates on the floor or lean them against equipment. Athletes return dumbbells to the rack in the proper order. They should not drop or throw weights or dumbbells.

7. Athletes should show respect for equipment and facilities at all times; spitting in or defacing the facility is not tolerated.

8. The weight room requires concentration. No horseplay, loud, offensive language, or temper tantrums.

9. The staff offices and telephones are off limits to athletes.

10. Wear proper training attire, particularly shirts and athletic shoes, at all times. No jeans or midriff shirts.

11. Use spotters when necessary.

12. Immediately report any facility-related injury or facility or equipment irregularity to the strength coach on duty.

13. Tobacco, food, chewing gum, glass bottles, cans, alcohol, drugs, and banned substances are not allowed in the lifting facility; plastic water bottles are acceptable.

14. Supervisors aren't responsible for users' personal belongings or lost or stolen items.

15. Keep feet off of the walls.

16. Minimize chalk and powder on the floor.

17. All guests and visitors must report to the office to sign liability forms and be approved to use the facility.

18. Former athletes using an athletic department weight room must have their program preapproved by a strength coach and must sign a release form.

19. Athletic department personnel can use these facilities for personal workouts if they don't interfere with the needs of the athletes.

20. Nonathletic department personnel are allowed to use the facilities with permission of the athletic director and after signing a waiver form. Recognized users include athletes, students, guests, staff, faculty with permission, former athletes, family members, and visiting teams.

21. No squatting outside the squat rack.

22. The on-duty supervisors have the authority over all weight room conduct and use of equipment and can expel an athlete from the facility for failure to follow instructions.

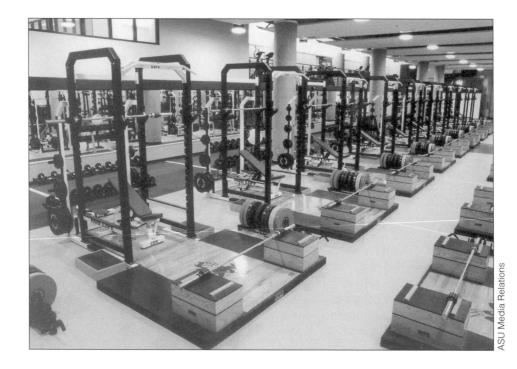

ARIZONA STATE

Strength coach Joe Kenn has put together a very impressive facility at Arizona State that features several four-post power racks from Power Lift. The four-post power racks come with adjustable bench/incline benches used inside the power rack. Joe chooses to use safety levels inside the power rack. These and the bar catch are manually adjustable. A pull-up attachment is mounted at the top of each power rack.

Explosive lifting is done on wooden platforms in front of the power racks. Wooden boxes are used to manually adjust the height of the bar for explosive lifting. Every major exercise can be done with this combination.

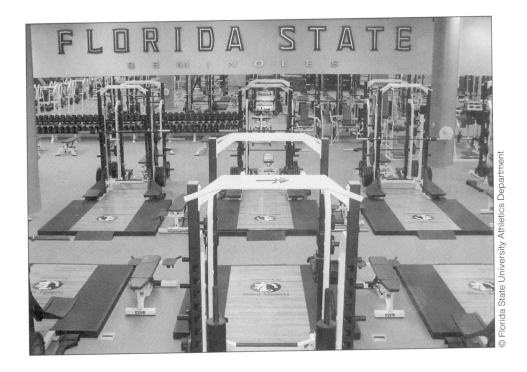

FLORIDA STATE UNIVERSITY

Strength coach Jon Jost takes a different approach to training his major exercises than that used at ASU. The Florida State facility also features Power Lift racks but uses the two-post half-racks rather than the four-post power racks. Jon prefers a row of dedicated half-racks used as bench/incline stations with adjustable bench/incline benches. No squats are done here even though the rack allows for them.

Another row of half-racks are provided for squats, and wooden platforms are provided in front of the half-racks for explosive lifting. For squatting, the bar height is adjusted manually with a bar catch while the technique trays serve as the safety level. The same technique trays are used to manually adjust the height of the bar for explosive lifting.

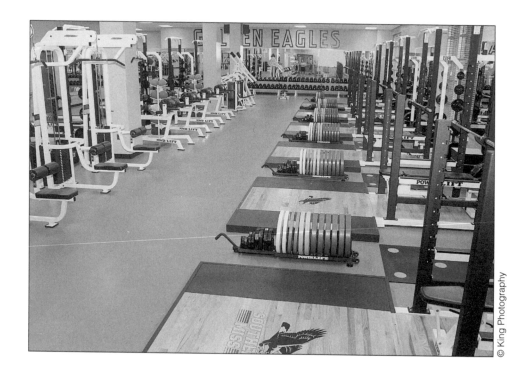

SOUTHERN MISSISSIPPI

Strength coach Charlie Dudley at Southern Mississippi uses yet another approach even though his facility is also equipped with Power Lift products. The Southern Mississippi facility features several four-post multi-racks with adjustable bench/incline benches used inside the multi-racks. Squats are done inside the multi-racks as safety levels and bar catches attached inside the multi-racks are manually adjustable.

Explosive lifting is done on wooden platforms in front of the multi-racks. Wooden boxes (not shown in this row of racks) are used to manually adjust the height of the bar for explosive lifting.

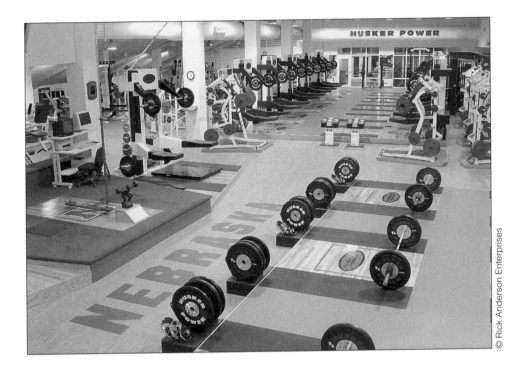

© Rick Anderson Enterprises

NEBRASKA

The Nebraska facility features several transformers similar to half-racks that mount on top of large wooden lifting platforms. The difference between the transformer and the half-rack is that the upper bar catch of the transformer moves to adjust the height of the bar electrically. The lower level also moves electrically and becomes the safety level for squats by moving up or down quickly. The transformers are used primarily for squats, hang cleans, and explosive overhead lifts, while bench and incline are done in Power Lift benches or incline stations made specifically for those exercises.

The lower arm of the transformer is used for the bar to rest on for hang cleans. A wooden platform is also provided in front of the transformer for power cleans.

Nebraska Facilities

Coaches and athletes visiting Nebraska facilities today probably think Nebraska athletes have always had whatever they wanted. That's not the case. Almost all of the equipment has been donated, even the air conditioning. It was 10 years before I got air conditioning in the weight room in the north fieldhouse. Stan Wentz, owner of Wentz Plumbing and Heating, happened to stop by the weight room in July and introduced himself. The heat was almost unbearable as the athletes lifted weights in preparation for fall camp. The excessive heat led Stan to collect 16 $1,000 donations from his associates to purchase two 10-ton air conditioning units.

Equipment innovations at Nebraska have had an impact on sports conditioning around the world. For many years, athletes were forced to use equipment designed and produced by manufacturers that seemed to have no regard for athletes. The equipment was designed to improve fitness, not build strength. Sometimes the weight stacks on machines wouldn't hold enough weight. Sometimes equipment wouldn't allow for tall athletes. American Manufacturing Foundry (AMF) changed all that when they asked me to design and endorse a line of strength and conditioning products for athletes in 1978. During the process, I came up with the hip sled for leg development on which athletes start out on their back and lift the weight with their legs. Almost every equipment company now has a version of the hip sled. I was looking for a way for I.M. Hipp, an All-American running back, to train his legs on a low-intensity workout day (called a "backoff day"). Hipp was squatting heavy, even on the mornings of football games and refused to miss his leg workouts. Needless to say, no one else in the country was doing heavy squats the morning of a football game. The hip sled didn't produce the gains the squat did because the board the athlete lay on provided most of the stabilization. But the hip sled also required less recovery, and in I.M. Hipp's case was helpful as a substitute for the squat.

The standing leg sled was a similar exercise done on the same apparatus, but some athletes could strain their back if they got their hips positioned too high. For Nebraska athletes, lying on the hip sled was more popular than using the leg sled. Joe Gitch, national sales manager for AMF American, flew me to their plant in Jefferson, Iowa, to make changes to the first prototype hip sled. They were calling it the EPR-150 (EPR stood for Epley Power Rack, and 150 was how much the carriage weighed). They later found out the EPR initials were already trademarked by someone else. Nebraska had been calling it the hip sled, and the name stuck.

Portable Weight Room

As Nebraska was preparing for the 1978 Orange Bowl, the bowl committee said they would provide lifting equipment at the bowl site. Prior to that, the team had no lifting during the 10 days at a bowl site. The Orange Bowl didn't realize what type of equipment or how much we needed. What they had for us wasn't sufficient. The Orange Bowl provided an old wobbly bench press bench and a 110 lb. barbell set. It wasn't an Olympic set but one like you might find in someone's basement after it rusted. I took a photo of the equipment they provided and vowed to bring my own equipment in the future. We were forced to take a bus to the Miami Dolphins' training facility after practice to lift weights that year.

For the 1980 Cotton Bowl, assistant strength coaches Mike Arthur and Gary Wade drove a van loaded with strength equipment and set up a portable weight room at the team's hotel. The problem with having the strength equipment at the hotel was doing laundry. The players' workout gear was all at the stadium and was cleaned each day between practices. At the hotel, the players had to wear their own personal clothes and had no way to launder them for the next day. Since then, Nebraska has upgraded to a 40,000-pound semi to haul its equipment to bowl games. We set up temporary weight rooms at the practice site, and laundry is no longer a problem. Lanny Fauss, owner of National Transportation, Inc., of Omaha was the first to donate his truck and driver (figure 6.4).

Wayne Tanderup's crew at Seward Motor Freight provided the service for several years. A contest was set up to determine the company's "safest driver." The winner's reward consisted of driving the Huskers' 15,000 pounds of strength equipment to their bowl game and back. One exception was the 2002 Rose Bowl, where the Huskers practiced, lifted, and ate at the University of Southern California. Crete Carrier started transporting the Huskers' bowl equipment in 2003. Many schools have

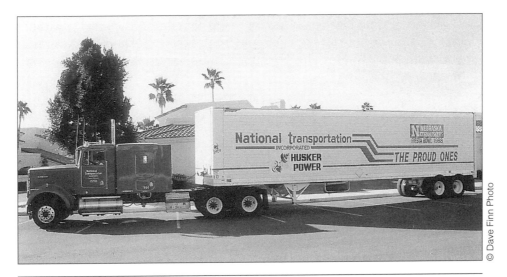

Figure 6.4 Nebraska was first to take equipment to bowl games with a semi-truck donated by National Transportation.

followed the lead and now take equipment to bowl games in semi-tractor trailers brightly painted with school logos.

Computerized Lifting Program

No one knew where to put the first Husker Power computer in 1978. My good friend Steve Pederson (now AD at Nebraska) suggested putting the computer on my desk. He told me, "You need to learn how to use it rather that rely on someone else in the future." Steve has always been a man with great vision, and he knew computers were going to take over in the future. It wasn't long before Husker Power had a computer on every strength coach's desk plus one in the weight room for the athletes to check their index points.

Nebraska was the first school in the country with computerized lifting programs for individual athletes. Mike Arthur and I then created a company to provide software for high school coaches. Mike was the driving force behind development of what we called the "Strength Disk," a lifting software program coaches could use to generate lifting programs for athletes. Many coaches still use the original Strength Disk software. In 2004, Husker Power created a new version of the Strength Disk (see strengthdisk.com).

Husker Power hired Daktronics in 1990 to install a computerized electronic sprint timer and scoreboard to display Performance Index points. When Nebraska athletes run the 10- and 40-yard dash, a computer collects all the data in six lanes at one time. Wires are run under the ground to and from each lane to a master computer. The only problem is the electronic times are about two-tenths of a second slower than hand-held times as the electronic timer starts immediately, rather than being delayed for the brief period of time it takes a human being to react to the start. Portable electronic timers were later developed by Randy Gobel and the Nebraska engineering department. The portable timers are used for indoor or outdoor use.

Equipment Innovations

Nebraska had a tremendous impact on strength-training equipment nationally in the '90s. Today almost every school uses equipment designed at Nebraska or copied from their designs. Husker Power hit back-to-back home runs with the development of the ground-based Jammer from Hammer Strength and the modular rack from Wynmor, then hit a grand slam with bases loaded with the design of the Nebraska transformer.

Hammer Jammer

The Jammer was developed by Gary Jones of the Hammer Strength Company and tested at Nebraska. It was the first of many ground-based pieces of equipment the company has successfully developed with my help. Hammer Strength was the leader in the country in making health club machines, and Nebraska had the reputation of being a free-weight facility, which was at the other end of the spectrum. The folks at Hammer Strength knew a lot of coaches looked to the University of Nebraska for leadership, so they were trying to bridge the gap by sending Nebraska one of their machines. The double incline was their top-selling machine until we explained the importance of the feet being on the ground for training. I asked Gary Jones if he could make machines with no seats on them. He invited me to his factory and agreed to make a prototype for Nebraska. He has since made several ground-based machines that have made a tremendous impact on how athletes train across the country. The Hammer Jammer soon became the number-one-selling machine in Hammer Strength history. Tom Proffitt, the national sales manager, said, "We found out what impact Boyd Epley and the Nebraska program had in the first year, when our dealers sold 54 Jammers across the rest of the nation while our Nebraska regional sales manager sold 250."

Modular Racks

I asked Gary Jones to develop a short power rack, but he was not interested (at least not in 1995). I then asked the Nebraska engineering department to help, but the drawing their students came up with wasn't what I wanted. We then hired Rick Lewis of Wynmor Fitness Systems in Topeka, Kansas, to develop the Husker Power Rack. Rick was the brother of Lance Lewis, who played fullback for the Huskers. Rick had just purchased a small equipment company and was looking for ways to get noticed. This rack led to modular training, which has revolutionized how racks are made and how weight rooms are designed in this country. Almost every equipment company now makes a rack with similar features. Modular racks can now be found in nearly every university program.

The Husker Power Rack evolved into a half-rack and then to a double-half-rack. The half-rack has two posts rather than four. Nebraska put eight of the double-half-racks in their facility. When Jeff Madden of Texas brought his board of regents to the Nebraska facility in 1998 and saw the racks, Madden went back to Texas and ordered 20 of them. Texas A&M bought 24, and many other universities also added the racks. Wynmor then added large wooden platforms to the racks, produced by Jeff Conner. Jeff was Hammer Strength's regional sales manager, but he was also building wooden inserts for Wynmor racks and selling both of these lines of equipment to high schools and colleges. I was under contract with Hammer Strength to endorse lever machines and to Wynmor to endorse modular racks. Both companies were creating products coaches needed and wanted, and Jeff Conner and I were involved with both.

Two big events happened in the same year that changed a few things for Jeff Conner and me. They also changed things for the strength industry and for anyone wanting to develop athletes. The first event was York Barbell's purchase of the small Wynmor company that was making those great racks. I had five years remaining on a contract with Wynmor to help create different versions of the racks. In a meeting with the York Barbell president, vice president, and national sales director for the division that would sell York's version of the racks, I was informed that York was not interested in my endorsement. I told them that I've always liked York Barbell and had great respect for all York had done for the strength industry. If they weren't interested in having me help, then the contract was done with as far as I was concerned. I only want to be involved with people who appreciate my help. York also had a division that made their own wooden inserts, which meant Jeff Conner was out as well. Jeff started Power Lift to make modular racks and wooden inserts and asked for my endorsement, which I was happy to give.

The Power Lift modular racks have now become the standard in the industry. Arizona State University was featured in *Sports Illustrated* in 2002 after installing 28 of them. Power Lift modular racks are being put in high schools and colleges all over the country. There appears to be a competition to see which school can squeeze in the most racks. Because Jeff was also the Hammer Strength regional director, he was able to cover the needs of a high school with racks or machines.

The other big event that affected the strength industry was the purchase of Hammer Strength by Life Fitness. Life Fitness made Hammer Strength part of a much larger dealer network with many more resources. Not only did Life Fitness want my endorsement, they sent engineers to Nebraska each year for input on new equipment concepts. The Life Fitness purchase gave Hammer Strength momentum to surge to the front of the strength industry—and because of Jeff Conner's affiliation, Power Lift surged to the front in the rack industry. As a consequence of all of this, the three men heading the York rack division when Jeff and I were helping them no longer work there, and York has discontinued its line of modular racks.

Husker Power Transformer

Nebraska put the rest of the nation on notice in 2002 with the design of the Husker Power Transformer. Husker Power is accustomed to taking a leadership position in the strength equipment field, but this time they're keeping it to themselves. Rivers Metal Products of Lincoln, Nebraska, was asked to design, develop, and install 14 custom-made transformers into the west stadium strength complex. The $25,000 machines give athletes who train with free weights unprecedented safety. The safety levels move electrically, which provides the most efficient way to train. Nebraska athletes have named the machine the "transformer" because it transforms from a squat machine into a hang clean machine with the touch of a button (figure 6.5). These all-electric machines also make for

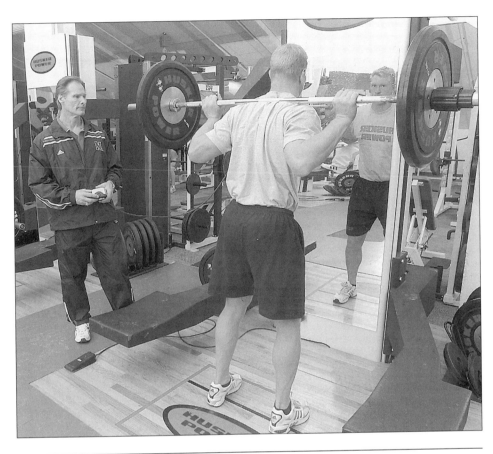

Figure 6.5   The Nebraska transformer provides a bar catch and safety level that adjusts up and down electrically.

the best environment for teaching proper lifting technique for both the explosive Olympic moves and the slower strength lifts.

Whether you are designing a facility from scratch or refurbishing an old one, take the time to work through the ten steps. It will take a little work, but you'll end up with a great facility based on the needs of your program.

Testing

7

In this chapter and the next three, we present a four-step process (testing, evaluating, goal setting, and program design) that can be used as a formula for success in any program, whether it's for an individual or a professional sport team. Any conditioning program should begin with the testing and evaluation of each participant. Once you have determined athletes' strengths and weaknesses, it's much easier to direct their training and achieve maximum results. Sports conditioning tests monitor progress on the components that contribute to the success of a given sport.

Testing also helps determine if a program is effectively achieving the desired goals. Do any athletes have obvious physical weaknesses? How are they progressing overall? These and many other questions can be answered through testing.

Another area in which testing is beneficial is in motivation. Many athletes, especially the younger ones, need positive proof that sports conditioning will benefit them before they're willing to put forth the effort to obtain maximum results. The key is to get your athletes to want to achieve new goals. Once they begin achieving goals, they'll be eager to set higher ones. It's always better to pull back on an athlete who is motivated rather than one who needs to be pushed. Pulling back on motivated athletes makes them hungrier; pulling back on underachievers reinforces their current attitudes.

Some schools overlook the tremendous benefits of the four-step process and begin lifting right away. Coaches who make the effort to test, evaluate, and set goals achieve results that can be documented.

Testing serves as a great motivator. At the end of one of our testing days for football players, when most of the players had finished, Heisman trophy winner Mike Rozier wasn't pleased with his time for the 40-yard dash. He asked for another run. I said okay, and when I looked up I couldn't help but notice he was stark naked. "Maybe I'll run faster in the nude," he said. We all got a big laugh out of it, but he didn't run any faster.

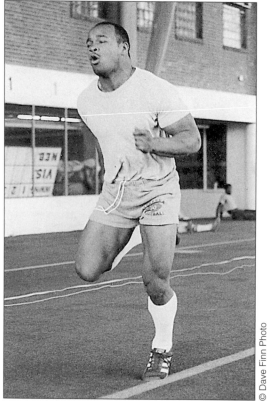

© Dave Finn Photo

Mike Rozier—dressed or undressed, equally fast.

Accurate Measurements

If not done properly, testing is meaningless for the coach and athlete. To ensure control, the coach should do the measurements, taking time for precise accuracy. Accurate measurements include *validity*, *reliability,* and *objectivity.*

Validity—each test must measure the component it is constructed to measure. Table 7.1 helps you determine the components associated with various tests.

Table 7.1 **Validity Table**	
Test	**Component**
Vertical jump	Lower body power
Pro agility	Agility
10-yard dash	Acceleration
40-yard dash	Speed
300-yard shuttle run	Conditioning

Reliability—testing conditions and measurement methods must be the same for each test. For example, testing results will differ if testing is done outside on grass one time, then inside on a basketball court another time. The condition of the field, time of day, and wind, rain, and temperature conditions all affect testing results.

Some factors are easily controlled, such as the testing order. The order in which the tests are done affects the results. For example, if you have your athletes run the 40-yard dash followed by the 300-yard shuttle during one testing period but run the 300-yard shuttle before the 40-yard dash during another period, the results of the 40-yard dash are guaranteed to be different. The testing order needs to be the same each and every time.

Testing equipment also needs to be the same each time. For example, the 40-yard dash can be done with electronic timers or with stopwatches. An electronically-timed 40-yard dash is usually about two tenths of a second higher on the average than a time measured with a stopwatch because the coach has to react to the start. The athlete starts to run, but the hand-held watch doesn't start recording until the coach can react; thus slightly less time is recorded. With electronic timing, the timer begins when the athlete starts running, therefore more time is recorded. Coaches have determined that hand-held times differ from electronic for big athletes about 2.4 tenths while smaller, faster athletes differ about 1.6 tenths.

Objectivity—to ensure consistent scoring, The same coaches should administer the same test each time, if possible. This will ensure more consistent scoring. If you must run a test with different coaches, be sure the test is administered in exactly the same way each time or it won't be reliable.

Annual Performance Test Cycle

The combination of testing periods form an annual test cycle, which ideally should take place during the week before a conditioning period starts. Testing establishes initial performance levels and determines the level of progress attained during the previous conditioning period. For a fall sport, the annual performance test cycle might be scheduled as follows.

Test Period Schedule

1. When athletes report in August
2. When the season is over in November or December
3. At the start of the postseason
4. After the off-season 12-week strength program

Performance Test Selection

When choosing performance tests, keep some simple guidelines in mind. The tests should be safe and easily administered. The athlete's frame of mind can affect the results of the test; lack of sleep can influence the testing results, as might personal problems, minor injuries, anxiety, or a temporary lack of motivation. These factors might be difficult to detect or prevent, but it can help to communicate with athletes before testing. Ask them if they feel ready to be tested, and if they say they don't, consider their reasons before moving ahead with the test. If appropriate, put the testing off for a short time.

The following tests are typical of the kind we do at Nebraska to measure athletes' body composition, power, lateral agility, speed, and conditioning.

Test 1: Height

The first body composition test involves measuring the athlete's height.

Materials Needed

- Flat wall against which the athlete stands
- Measuring tape or marked area on wall
- Device to place on the head of the athlete that forms a right angle with the wall

Procedure

1. Athlete takes off shoes.
2. Athlete stands with heels, buttocks, back, and head against the wall.

3. Place device on the athlete's head so that a right angle is formed with the wall.
4. Measure to the nearest half-inch and record height.

Causes for Disqualification
- Not having shoes off
- Not having feet flat on the floor and buttocks against the wall

Test 2: Body Weight

The second test for determining body composition involves measuring the athlete's body weight.

Materials Needed
Certified scale

Procedure
1. Athlete must weigh in wearing only a T-shirt, shorts, and socks (no shoes, sweats, or equipment).
2. Athlete should weigh in before any activity to avoid fluctuations caused by dehydration.
3. Round body weight to the nearest whole pound.

Causes for Disqualification
- Inappropriate attire
- Attempting to increase body weight by attaching a weight to the body

Test 3: Waist Circumference

In addition to height and body weight, include a waist-circumference measurement to monitor changes in body composition.

Materials Needed
Flexible tape measure (cloth or vinyl)

Procedure
1. Athlete should stand relaxed with arms at sides.
2. Measurement should be taken with tape around waist at navel height.
3. Tape measure should be pulled until taut but not stretched or twisted.
4. Record to the nearest quarter-inch.

Test 4: Vertical Jump

The vertical jump (with Vertec) measures power, which refers to an athlete's ability to apply maximum force as quickly as possible. Power relates to a player's ability to make the quick, explosive movements necessary for success in most sports. If you're going to use only one test for your athletes, make it the vertical jump. It's the best indicator of talent.

Materials Needed

- Area marked on wall in half-inch intervals
- Vertec testing device
- Adjustment rod

Procedure

1. Athlete stands with one side to the wall.
2. Make sure feet and hips are next to the wall.
3. Athlete reaches as high as possible, keeping feet flat on the floor.
4. Record the height reached to the nearest half-inch.
5. The athlete then goes to the Vertec and positions feet flat (figure 7.1a).
6. The athlete then jumps, hitting the highest possible line on the Vertec (figure 7.1b). No steps are taken before the jump.
7. Record the height jumped to the nearest half-inch.
8. Subtract the height reached from the height jumped.
9. Record the better of the two trials.

Example: Height jumped (124 inches) minus height reached (94 inches) equals a vertical jump of 30 inches. Record the total number of inches the athlete jumped in the box marked "jump" in the chart provided on page 148. Under "score," record the difference between the height reached and the height jumped to the nearest half-inch. Record the vertical jump score and give the athlete feedback right at the testing site. Go to huskerpower.com and click the coaches menu option to see the vertical jump calculation to determine index points. Enter the athlete's weight and how high he or she jumped to calculate vertical jump index points.

Causes for Disqualification

- Not having feet and hips next to the wall when reaching
- Standing on tiptoes when reaching
- Taking a step before the jump
- Taking a shuffle jump before jumping

Tables 7.2–7.4 show the vertical jump statistics for various athletes.

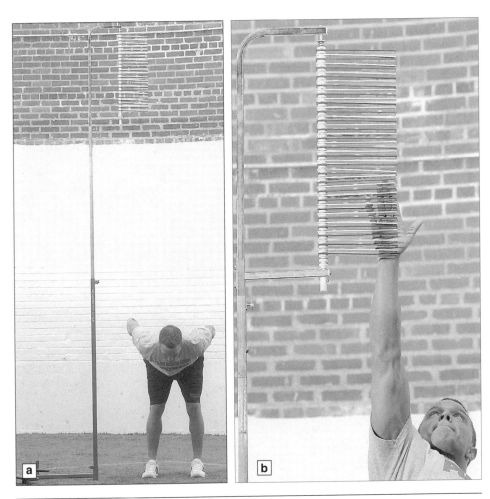

Figure 7.1 *(a)* The athlete prepares for the vertical jump. *(b)* The Vertec plastic vanes identify the height of the jump.

Table 7.2 Nebraska Vertical Jump Records

All-time records	Jump (inches)	Name	Year
Women	30	Peaches James	2001
Men	41.5	Trev Alberts	1994
Football	**Jump**	**Name**	**Year**
Rush ends	41.5	Trev Alberts	1994
Defensive backs	41	Curtin Cotton	1989
I-backs	41	James Sims	1996
Wide receivers	40	Dana Brinson	1987
Linebackers	40	Jamel Williams	1996

(continued)

Table 7.2 *(continued)*

Football	Jump	Name	Year
Offensive line	39.5	Keven Lightner	1985
Fullbacks	38.5	Curt Tomasevicz	2001
Defensive tackles	36.5	Kenny Walker	1989
Quarterbacks	36.5	Jay Runty	1999
Tight ends	36	Johnny Mitchell	1990
Track	**Jump**	**Name**	**Year**
Men	40	Chris Chandler	2000
Women	29.5	Angee Henry	1996
Baseball/softball	**Jump**	**Name**	**Year**
Men	38.5	John Cole	2000
Women	30	Peaches James	2001
Basketball	**Jump**	**Name**	**Year**
Men	37	Ross Buckendahl	2001
Women	26.5	Tanya Upthegrove	1994
Wrestling	**Jump**	**Name**	**Year**
Men	33.5	Ryan Schultz	1998
Tennis	**Jump**	**Name**	**Year**
Men	30	Fungai Tongoona	2000
Women	24	Ndali Ijomah	2000
Volleyball	**Jump**	**Name**	**Year**
Women	28	Laura Pilakowski	2001
Soccer	**Jump**	**Name**	**Year**
Women	26.5	Kori Saunders	2001

Table 7.3 Vertical Jump Averages

NCAA football	Jump (inches)
Split ends, strong safeties, backs	31.5
Wide receivers, outside linebackers	31
Linebackers, tight ends, safeties	29.5
Quarterbacks	28.5
Defensive tackles	28
Offensive guards	27
Offensive tackles	25.5

Men	Jump (inches)
NCAA basketball	28
NCAA baseball	23
High school football backs and ends	24
College recreational	24
NCAA tennis	23
High school football linebackers	22
High school football linemen	20
17-year-old boys	20
18- to 36-year-old men	16
Women	**Jump (inches)**
NCAA basketball	21
Competitive college athletes	18.5
NCAA tennis	15
College recreational	15
17-year-old girls	13
18- to 34-year-old women	8

Data from NSCA Essentials of Strength and Conditioning, 2nd Ed. (Baechle and Earle, editors), 2000, Human Kinetics.

Table 7.4 NFL Combined Vertical Jump Data

Position	Best jump	Average
Quarterbacks	38.5	32.5
Running backs	42	35
Wide receivers	41.5	36.5
Tight ends	38.5	33
Offensive line	37.5	32
Defensive tackles	34.5	31
Defensive ends	40.5	34.5
Linebackers	42	35
Defensive backs	41	35.5

Test 5: Pro Agility Run

The Pro Agility Run measures lateral agility, which is the ability to change directions rapidly while maintaining balance without losing any speed. Record the average of two runs.

Athletes can do this test from a standing start or a three-point start as long as everyone on the team does it the same way. The NFL starts with the hand down. The athlete runs to the left for 5 yards, then returns running 10 yards to the right before coming back to the starting line (figure 7.2). The total distance run is 20 yards. The Nebraska portable timer has a built-in delay that allows the athlete to cross the beam the first time without stopping the timer. As the athlete crosses the beam again, the agility time is displayed. If hand-held stopwatches are used, record the average time from two coaches.

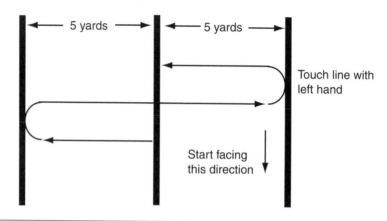

Figure 7.2 Pro agility run.

Tests 6 and 7: 10-Yard Dash and 40-Yard Dash

These tests measure acceleration and speed. The number-one physical attribute that determines athletic ability is running speed. A fast start and good acceleration are very important; being a step faster could be the difference between winning and losing.

Materials Needed

- Portable electronic timer (without electronic timing, the 10-yard time will not be accurate enough to record)
- 60 yards of flat running surface

Procedure

1. Stretching and warming up properly is of extreme importance.
2. Athlete places one hand on the starting line.
3. Athlete starts when ready. The timer starts automatically when the athlete's hand leaves the start switch.
4. Record the best time in the "score column" of figure 7.5 (page 148).

Test 8: 300-Yard Shuttle Run

The 300-yard shuttle run measures conditioning, which can be the deciding factor toward the end of many athletic competitions. You don't need to include this test in every testing session, but it should be done before the start of each competitive season.

Materials Needed

- Five stopwatches
- One measured course (25 yards with two lanes)
- Three coaches or managers
- Recording charts (and clipboards)

Procedure

1. Stretch and warm up before beginning one of two trials.

2. Two athletes line up in the first trial lane and start on the timer's command (each timer has two watches).

3. The athletes sprint the 25-yard course and back to the starting line for six round trips (12 × 25 yards equals 300 yards). See figure 7.3.

4. Foot contact must be made on the starting line and the 25-yard line each time when changing directions.

5. On completion of the first trial, the rest timer starts the watch to measure the five minutes between the athlete's first and second trials. The athlete(s) may walk or stretch but must be ready to start the second trial after a five-minute rest.

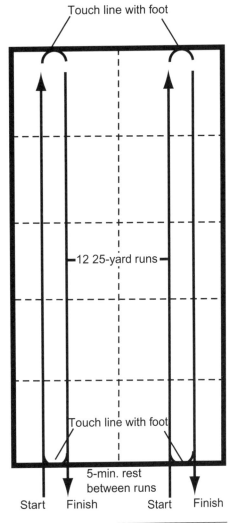

Figure 7.3 300-yard shuttle run.

6. The timer in the first trial can start another pair of athletes about a minute after the first pair has completed their first trial. It's the responsibility of the timer in the first lane to tell the rest timer when a group has completed a trial so that the rest time can be started. The rest timer need not ever stop his or her watch but just record the time on a piece of

paper and add five minutes to that time. When the five minutes is up, the rest timer tells the timer of the second trial lane to start the athletes on their second run.

7. After the two trials are complete, there should be two times recorded to the nearest 10th of a second. The average of the two times should also be recorded (e.g., if the first run is 52.4 seconds and the second run is 56.6 seconds, the average is 54.5 seconds).

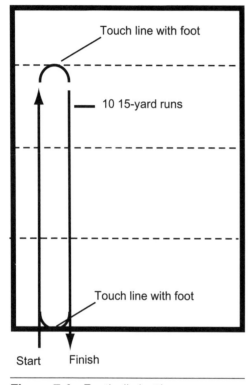

Touch line with foot

10 15-yard runs

Touch line with foot

Start   Finish

Figure 7.4 Football shuttle run.

Note: It's important to look at the difference between the two times. Athletes in very poor physical condition will have trouble on the second run (e.g., 58 seconds first run, 70 seconds second run). Averaging the two times might have to be done after the testing period has been completed if there's not enough time during the on-site testing.

The 300-yard shuttle works better for basketball than football. In 2002, we changed the test for football to 10 round trips of 15 yards in place of 6 round trips of 25 yards (see figure 7.4). This change provided more stops and turns and increased the number of times the player had to accelerate. The test was also reduced to one run in contrast to the standard method of running it again after a five-minute recovery period. Running only once made the test much shorter in total time but more intense. Nebraska found the shorter test yielded all the information needed about conditioning for football.

Steps for Administering a Test

Planning ahead is essential for any testing program. For accurate results and a smooth testing session, your testing equipment, facilities, personnel assignments, and test instructions must all be organized in advance. To help you get organized, follow the following steps.

Before Test Day

1. Schedule the test. Scheduling the test period might involve meeting with the coaches assigned to help in addition to meeting with the athletes to explain essential procedures.

2. Organize the equipment and facility. The more you do in advance, the smoother your testing day will go. Determine the equipment and facilities you'll need and get them ready. First, get permission to use the facility at the time you need it. Then secure all the equipment and make sure everything is in working order and calibrated. Also make sure that your facilities have enough space to conduct each test safely for the number of athletes you're testing. You might want to draw a floor plan to help you organize the testing stations. Use the floor plan to show athletes how traffic should flow as they move from one station to another. Be sure the athletes have enough space to slow down after running. Also ensure that there's enough traction to run without falling down or slipping. Look at each test and give thought to any potential hazards. It's your responsibility to avoid injuries in your athletes. If a serious injury does occur, chances are very good that a court of law will determine if you have acted within the standards of your profession.

   Next, you'll want to estimate the time needed for testing. If this is your first testing session, you might want to allow extra time. Estimating the time in advance minimizes confusion and maximizes the use of the time available.

3. Recruit volunteers to help. You might want to recruit some help with the testing session. Usually, other coaches are the most reliable help. If you don't have the manpower to put one person at each test station, you might have to test the whole group on one test, and then move the entire group to the next test.

4. Notify athletes. The next step is to develop a test schedule for the athletes and post it for athletes to see. The schedule should include the date and time of the test, who will be taking it, where it will be held, and what tests will be required. It's also a good idea to post your floor plan, so that athletes have advance directions on how to move from one station to the next.

5. Develop data collection cards. Have your athletes carry data collection cards with them to each station, on which the supervisor records test results. Using cards is easier than posting a roster at each station. The card should include all the tests being administered and personal information such as the athlete's name and the date. List the tests in the order in which they're to be performed. This way the athletes can use the cards as a plan to follow. A sample data collection card is shown in figure 7.5.

On Test Day

1. Warm up. There are two types of warm-ups. General warm-up is the basic stretching routine used to warm up athletes for a practice or game. Specific warm-up is done by performing the actual test at

Performance Test Data Collection Card

Your school's logo

Test date _____

Athlete's name _____

Position _____ Height _____

Body weight _____ Waist _____

Test	Performance		Score
Pro agility	Right	Left	Average
Vertical jump	Reach	Jump	
10-yard dash	First	Second	Best
40-yard dash	First	Second	Best
300-yard shuttle run	First		

Figure 7.5 Sample performance test data collection card.

submaximal speed or effect. Allow athletes a few warm-up trials on their own off to the side without being scored.

2. Announce scores. After the athlete executes each test, announce the score right away. This gives immediate feedback and also motivates athletes to give their best effort. At Nebraska, we actually record the athlete's best effort on the testing card for each test session.

3. Notice any traffic flow problems. Are there any bottlenecks or waiting lines? If a problem can't be corrected during this testing session, make sure you correct it next time. You might need more equipment or more volunteers.

4. Collect testing cards. The coach or volunteer at the last station collects all the cards. Make sure everyone has completed each test and recorded all necessary information.

Annual Strength Test Cycle

Strength levels can be taken during a lifting workout or, to motivate athletes, can be done within a testing format. Refer to the Big Picture, presented in chapter 10, to determine when to test strength levels. For fall sports, you should check strength level at the end of the base phase around week 13. Have your athletes lift as much weight as they can for 5 to 6 reps for explosive lifts and up to 10 reps for strength movements. Check strength level again at the end of the development phase in week 17 by lifting as much as possible for 3 to 4 reps for explosive and 3 to 5 reps for strength movements. Another strength level should be taken after the peak phase, around week 21, by doing 1 to 2 reps on explosive and 1 to 3 on strength movements. Strength testing is a little different than measuring strength levels in a workout. For motivation, strength testing is sometimes handled more like a lifting meet. You can use the sample card in figure 7.6 to record the strength test data.

We recommend doing your strength testing just before the playing season starts. Have athletes lift as much weight as they can for 1 to 2 reps on explosive lifts and 1 to 3 on strength movements. Then go to the huskerpower.com Web site to enter the poundage lifted and number of reps to calculate the 1RM. If you join the Members Only club, you can also enter an athlete's body weight and get index points so that athletes can compete with each other. Index points are explained in detail in chapter 8. The Nebraska strength complex has a 100-inch video screen just above the record platform that allows athletes to see their points as they lift so they know how many repetitions they need to score the desired index points.

Be sure to check out how the Members Only section on huskerpower.com can help you enter your test data and compare one athlete to another as you track their progress year to year. Testing can serve as a great motivator if done correctly.

Strength Test Data Collection Card

Your school's logo

Test date _____

Athlete's name _____

Position _____ Height _____

Body weight _____ Waist _____

Test	Strength		Score
Hang clean	lbs	reps	1RM
Bench press	lbs	reps	1RM
Squat	lbs	reps	1RM

Figure 7.6 Sample strength test data collection card.

8

Evaluation

The data from performance testing and strength testing should be compiled each test period into a format that enables the coach to interpret the test scores and evaluate how the team and each person is progressing. The best way to do this is to create team and individual profiles. Looking at team averages for each category on a team performance profile or a team strength profile allows coaches to see how athletes performed as a team during a particular period.

Team Performance and Strength Profiles

Comparing athletes' current testing averages to previously set goals and past team averages reveals strengths and weaknesses in your sports conditioning program and lets you know how effective the program has been. For example, you might see progress in strength but no progress in the areas of speed and power. This information tells you what adjustments need to be made in the program for this particular group of athletes. See tables 8.1 and 8.2 for sample team performance and team strength profiles.

In this team performance profile example, the group average was 2,306 points. By comparing this number and the individual category averages along the bottom of the chart to the group results from the previous year, you can quickly see progress made. In addition to the name and position, height and weight

Table 8.1 Team Performance Profile

Performance Report—Football—03/10/2000

Football test

Name	Position	Ht	Wt	10	10 pts.
Alexander	Running back	5-11.25	251	1.62	754
Vanden Bosch	Rush end	6-4	268	1.67	713
Bauman	Tight end	6-2	262	1.65	733
Buckhalter	Running back	5-11.5	229	1.65	571
Baker	Linebacker	6-0	234	1.60	694
Kasier	Defensive line	6-4	288	1.75	638
Kosch	Receiver	5-9.5	192	1.62	497
Ryan	Rush end	6-0.75	233	1.69	540
Schwab	Offensive line	6-1.25	299	1.75	675
Grummert	Rush end	6-2	242	1.69	587
Bender	Receiver	5-11	185	1.61	470
List	Defensive back	5-11	219	1.74	410
Anderson	Defensive back	5-8	173	1.59	470
Hochstein	Offensive line	6-3.75	280	1.78	556
Woodward	Defensive back	5-7.5	178	1.63	433
Sherman	Offensive line	6-4	299	1.80	587
Ortiz	Linebacker	6-0.5	221	1.73	433
Beveridge	Receiver	6-0	191	1.68	421
Watchorn	Defensive back	5-10.75	198	1.63	497
Buettenback	Linebacker	5-11.25	220	1.71	445
Session averages:			233	1.68	556

40	40 pts.	PRO	PRO pts.	VJump	VJump pts.	P Index
4.53	968	3.96	893	31.5	530	3,145
4.78	744	4.07	850	34.5	632	2,939
4.80	704	4.11	788	35.5	663	2,888
4.61	754	3.88	810	37.0	692	2,827
4.74	647	4.12	605	35.0	625	2,571
5.21	477	4.22	751	29.0	492	2,358
4.76	519	3.75	839	31.0	471	2,326
4.93	497	4.02	695	31.5	519	2,251
5.19	533	4.34	662	23.5	375	2,245
4.90	548	4.17	614	29.0	459	2,208
4.66	579	3.94	618	33.5	527	2,194
4.85	511	3.92	735	31.5	511	2,167
4.73	511	3.98	561	36.0	590	2,132
5.20	445	4.23	710	24.5	379	2,090
4.59	630	4.12	472	33.5	522	2,057
5.23	504	4.51	523	26.0	428	2,042
4.82	548	4.15	546	31.5	513	2,040
4.81	484	3.91	672	30.5	459	2,036
4.84	471	3.99	614	28.5	417	1,999
5.20	315	4.24	472	26.0	381	1,613
4.87	569	4.08	672	31.0	509	2,306

Table 8.2 Team Strength Profile

Strength Report—Football—03/10/2000

Football test

Name	Position	Ht	Wt	CI	CI pts.	Sq	Sq pts.	S Index
Alexander	Running back	5-11.25	251	330	447	450	424	871
Vanden Bosch	Rush end	6-4	268	363	500	560	514	1,014
Bauman	Tight end	6-2	262	357	494	478	440	934
Buckhalter	Running back	5-11.5	229	236	301	350	363	664
Baker	Linebacker	6-0	234	363	580	450	439	1,019
Kasier	Defensive line	6-4	288	363	461	490	435	896
Kosch	Receiver	5-9.5	192	330	577	480	509	1,086
Ryan	Rush end	6-0.75	233	360	571	562	550	1,121
Schwab	Offensive line	6-1.25	299	363	442	690	646	1,088
Grummert	Rush end	6-2	242	363	556	475	454	1,010
Bender	Receiver	5-11	185	335	619	457	517	1,136
List	Defensive back	5-11	219	368	635	523	523	1,158
Anderson	Defensive back	5-8	173	187	298	370	463	761
Hochstein	Offensive line	6-3.75	280	363	481	505	452	933
Woodward	Defensive back	5-7.5	178	368	753	523	610	1,363
Sherman	Offensive line	6-4	299	372	464	559	496	960
Ortiz	Linebacker	6-0.5	221	330	508	433	432	940
Beveridge	Receiver	6-0	191	303	500	350	392	892
Watchorn	Defensive back	5-10.75	198	291	459	430	450	909
Buettenback	Linebacker	5-11.25	220	329	516	503	502	1,018
Session averages:			233	333.7	508	481.9	481	989

are listed. The recommended tests are the 10-yard dash time, followed by the index score for the 10-yard dash. This index takes into account what the athlete weighs to calculate the index. You could sort this group by position to see how the position such as the offensive line did this test period as compared to last test period. The 40-yard dash time is also followed by the index as are the pro agility run and vertical jump. The final column is the total index, which adds the four performance index scores together. Any individual scores over 500 are very good. A T-shirt is awarded for posting all four index scores over 500. Only five athletes achieved that in this example.

The team strength profile is very similar except there are only two tests that make up the strength index, the clean and the squat. Coaches who use the index points soon learn that an increase in strength will increase the performance profile, which results in an automatic improvement in athletic performance.

Individual Performance and Strength Profiles

Of course, you'll also want to evaluate your athletes individually. With individual profiles, it's important to keep a history of each athlete's testing because performance scores from a single test period never tell the whole story. Good records allow you and the athlete's coaches to evaluate the progress the athlete has made from one year to the next. Almost always, athletes progress most during their first year of training. Each succeeding year, less progress is made as athletes approach their athletic potential.

Focus on making progress in the areas in which the athlete has weaknesses. The individual profile is particularly useful for one-on-one conferences with athletes. Note at the bottom of the individual profiles shown in tables 8.3 and 8.4 that you can see the athlete's best performance (high scores). We use this feature to motivate athletes during performance tests. We print their best score on the test card so that they have it with them when they're testing. In Nebraska's football program, if a senior scores a personal best on any test, he doesn't have to run the 300-yard shuttle run. A junior must improve on two tests to avoid the shuttle run, and a sophomore must improve on three. New freshmen all have to run the 300-yard shuttle to demonstrate they can achieve the minimum standard time required to participate in the sport. With this reward system in place, athletes take testing seriously and give a focused effort on each test. In fact, they sometimes beg for additional attempts if they're just short of their personal best.

Table 8.3   Individual Performance Profile

Performance Report—Gregg List

Date	Ht	Wt	10	10 pts.	40
8/11/2002	5-11	212	1.72	421	
3/19/2002	5-11	198.4	1.67	445	4.68
1/20/2002	5-11	225	1.66	526	4.91
8/7/2002	5-11	222	1.71	458	
3/18/2002	5-11	219.4	1.66	511	4.69
1/26/2002	5-11	217	1.66	511	4.78
8/8/2002	5-11	211	1.68	470	
3/10/2002	5-11	219	1.74	410	4.85
1/27/2002	5-11	196	1.66	458	4.74
High scores:			1.66	526	4.68

Table 8.4   Individual Strength Profile

Strength Report—Gregg List

Date	Ht	Wt	Cl	Cl pts.	Sq	Sq pts.	S Index
8/11/2002	5-11	212					
3/19/2002	5-11	198.4	297	474	488	505	979
1/20/2002	5-11	225					
8/7/2002	5-11	222					
3/18/2002	5-11	219.4	336	536	475	475	1,011
1/26/2002	5-11	217	346	565	520	520	1,085
8/8/2002	5-11	211					
3/10/2002	5-11	219	368	635	523	523	1,158
1/27/2002	5-11	196					
High scores:			368	635	523	523	1,158

Performance Index

In the late 1970s, an interest developed in identifying an athlete's overall athletic aptitude. Nebraska has analyzed over 20,000 cases of Division I athletic performances and developed a testing methodology that measures baseline athletic aptitude along a standardized point scale, controlling for weight. The tests Nebraska uses correlate with on-field performance. They have been included in a composite indicator we call the Performance Index, which is a general indicator of potential performance. Although other elements significantly contribute to on-field performance (such as the practice field work habits of a Jerry Rice, the game-day heart of a Michael Jordan, the level of skill development of a Pete Rose, and the intangible intuitive feel for the game of a Larry Bird), we find the performance index to be a very useful instrument in identifying raw athletic talent. Of course there's no guarantee that, once identified, this raw talent will be exhibited on the playing field. Rather, like an ACT or SAT college exam score, the Performance Index reveals baseline athletic talents and indicates who is *likely* to do well. The primary features of our Performance Index are listed here.

Performance Index Features

- The index is based on a decathlon-type scoring system in which athletes receive points based on performance. The higher they jump,

40 pts.	PRO	PRO pts.	VJump	VJump pts.	P Index
	4.36	391	29.5	454	1,266
587	4.15	492	32.0	502	2,026
484	4.04	635	28.0	426	2,071
	4.01	662	29.5	461	1,581
638	4.05	614	30.5	484	2,247
564	4.14	542	28.5	435	2,052
	3.98	662	28.5	430	1,562
511	3.92	735	31.5	511	2,167
541	4.08	542	28.5	417	1,958
638	3.92	735	32.0	511	2,247

the more points they receive. The faster they run, the more points they receive.

- The index is scored on a 0- to 1,000-point system for each event. The index has been standardized so that a score of 500 is considered a solid, NCAA Division I performance standard that is not easy to achieve.
- The index, developed for both genders, includes the vertical jump, the agility run, the 10-yard dash, and the 40-yard dash. These scores are then combined for an overall score.
- The index controls for weight differences among athletes in an attempt to identify, pound for pound, the fastest, most powerful athlete. Lighter athletes are expected to run faster in the running events. For example, to receive an index score of 500 points, a 275-pound athlete must run the 40-yard dash in roughly 5 seconds. For a 200-pound athlete to receive an index score of 500 points, he must run the 40-yard dash in 4.8 seconds. In other words, the index is internally consistent.
- The index is also externally consistent. In other words, after analyzing 20,000 cases over 25 years, Nebraska has concluded that 500 points on the vertical jump is equivalent to 500 points on the 10-yard dash, which is equivalent to 500 points in the agility run, and so on.
- The index uses NCAA Division I championship performances and world records as the basis of its standardization.
- The nature of the point system is such that athletes receive more points the closer they get to the ultimate performance. For instance, if a 200-pound athlete improved his vertical jump from 10 inches to 11 inches, he would receive approximately 2 points, but if another 200-pound athlete improved his vertical jump from 34 to 35 inches,

Table 8.5 Three-Person Sample Performance Profile

Performance Report—Football—03/10/2000

Football test

Name	Position	Ht	Wt	10	10 pts.
List	Defensive back	5-11	219	1.74	410
Woodward	Defensive back	5-7.5	178	1.63	433
Watchorn	Defensive back	5-10.75	198	1.63	497
Session averages:			198	1.67	447

he would receive approximately 50 points. The second athlete's achievement is much more significant than the first athlete's and is scored accordingly.

- The index is an instructional tool. By examining the scores received for the various tests, athletes and coaches can easily see which areas need the most improvement.

We use the Strength Index in the same ways we use the Performance Index except that different skills are tested. The strength tests include the squat and hang clean; the two tests are combined for an overall score. See tables 8.5 and 8.6 for examples of three athletes' performance and strength profiles as determined by the indexes.

Consider the information shown in tables 8.5 and 8.6 to quickly evaluate the strengths and weaknesses of the three athletes. For instance, Troy Watchorn ran the 10-yard dash in 1.63 seconds. For Watchorn's weight class (198 pounds), this performance received a score of 497 points. Watchorn also scored nearly 500 in the 40-yard dash (471 points) for his 4.84 time, and his agility run netted 614 points. He wasn't quite as good on the vertical jump, scoring 417 points for a jump of 28.5 inches. If you look at the scores from each test (497, 471, 614, 417), you see right away with the 614 agility score that Watchorn has exceptional change of direction. You might think he needs to focus his efforts on generating more power to improve his vertical jump. But when you note his strength index scores of 435 points for the hang clean and 450 for the squat, you see that Troy is actually a pretty well-balanced athlete without any glaring weakness.

Note that Gregg List, who ran nearly the same 40 time as Watchorn (4.85) but weighed 20 pounds more, received 511 points for the 40-yard dash versus 471 for Troy. They ran the same time, but List received more points because he weighed more. The strength index is just the opposite. List weighed 219 and cleaned 368 pounds for 635 points, whereas Wes

40	40 pts.	PRO	PRO pts.	VJump	VJump pts.	P Index
4.85	511	3.92	735	31.5	511	2,167
4.59	630	4.12	472	33.5	522	2,057
4.84	471	3.99	614	28.5	417	1,999
4.76	537	4.01	607	31.2	483	2,074

Table 8.6 Three-Person Sample Strength Profile

Strength Report—Football—03/10/2000

Football test

Name	Position	Ht	Wt	CI	CI pts.	Sq	Sq pts.	S Index
List	Defensive back	5-11	219	368	635	523	523	1,158
Woodward	Defensive back	5-7.5	178	368	753	420	496	1,249
Watchorn	Defensive back	5-10.75	198	281	435	430	450	885
Session averages:			198	339	608	457.7	490	1,097

Woodward scored 753 points for lifting the same poundage (368) at a body weight of 178.

The Performance Index is not only a solid indicator of potential on-field performance but also a powerful motivational tool. Athletes of different sizes and even in different sports compete with one another as they strive for the same goal of 500 (or more) points on the various tests. It takes little time for athletes to understand that 500 points is 500 points, regardless of the event and body size. There is a significant amount of mutual support and understanding as the athletes work together toward achieving this common goal. In our sample group shown in the tables, the team averages are all above the 500-point level except for the squat, the 10-yard dash, and the vertical jump. A good goal for this group would be to achieve above 500 points on all tests for the next test period.

The Performance Index helps athletes of various sizes quantitatively see where they stand compared to their peers in raw athletic aptitude. This information has proven to be extremely useful in helping athletes and coaches set realistic goals in moving to the next level of performance capability.

The Performance Index can also be used to measure the effectiveness of overall conditioning programs and serve as a warning of possible overtraining.

Nebraska has used the Performance Index for over 25 years as an integral part of its male and female athletic programs. We should again emphasize, however, that though the index can serve as a solid indicator of raw athletic aptitude and motivate athletes in their workout programs, it does not measure the drive, determination, and technical skills necessary for optimal achievement on the field or court.

The six tests used for the Performance Index and Strength Index can't be included in book form because they require a computer to make a series of calculations. One of the tests, the vertical jump, is provided free of charge on the huskerpower.com Web site. After many requests for access to index points for all six tests, we have created a Members Only section on the site. Members have access to the Performance Index (10-yard dash, 40-yard dash, vertical jump, and agility run) and the Strength Index (squat and hang clean). The points for the bench press are also included on the Strength Index, but Nebraska no longer uses the bench press in their total scoring. If you have any questions or comments while you're looking over the Web site, call us at 402-472-3333. We'll answer your questions and tell you how to be a part of our Members Only club.

Once each year Nebraska takes a photo of current athletes who have achieved Record Platform status. This honor is available to all athletes. Athletes must score 500 or more points on all six tests to be included on the Record Platform. Table 8.7 shows Nebraska's record Performance Index scores.

The Performance Index scores are used by Nebraska coaches to evaluate high school athletes who attend our summer camps. The Nebraska Football School, for example, has over 1,800 athletes each summer in four sessions. On average for each year, fewer than 10 athletes attending the camps score over 2,000 Performance Index points.

Measuring Intensity

Strength coaches tend to evaluate how athletes are doing in the weight room based on attendance, but attendance alone won't identify those who are or are not getting the job done. In 1997, Nebraska learned the importance of intensity. We had perfect attendance the first few weeks of the season but noticed that our normal hard workers weren't lifting as much weight as they normally did. Scott Frost, the starting quarterback, who was capable of doing 300 pounds for 10 reps on the hang clean, was using an unusually light weight. We informed the football coaches that the players were coming into the weight room exhausted after being overtrained at practice. Coach Osborne reduced the demands of practice and put in additional rest breaks, and this corrected the problem. We then instituted a grading system to be sure our players were working at the proper intensity in the weight room. The athlete was given a 2 if he did the correct lift with the recommended amount of weight. If he used too light a poundage on the lift, he got a 1. If he didn't do the lift or did a lesser exercise instead, he got a 0. Position grades were calculated and averaged, and an offense versus defense grade was shown to the players each week.

The key to this grading system is to identify major lifts that would generate a 2 grade if done correctly. For us, the squat is a 2, but someone

Table 8.7 Nebraska School Record Index Chart

All-time Nebraska Performance Index records		Points	Year
James Sims	Football	3,313	1996
Laura Pilakowski	Volleyball	2,394	2002
Football records by position			
IB	James Sims	3,313	1996
DB	Curtis Cotton	3,227	1991
FB	Dan Alexander	3,144	1998
RU	Kyle Vanden Bosch	2,939	1999
TE	Johnny Mitchell	2,909	1991
LB	Brian Shaw	2,817	1997
DL	Jon Clanton	2,788	1999
OL	Freddy Pollack	2,779	1996
REC	Nate Turner	2,765	1991
QB	Scott Frost	2,686	1996
KP	Bill Lafleur	2,423	1998
Other sports records			
Baseball	Ken Harvey	2,627	1998
Men's Basketball	Cookie Belcher	2,537	2000
Volleyball	Laura Pilakowski	2,394	2002
Women's Basketball	Margaret Richards	2,294	2000
Soccer	Julie Greco	2,218	1997
Softball	Anne Steffan	2,178	2002
Women's Track & Field	Shelley Ann Brown	2,096	2002
Wrestling	Tolly Thompson	1,804	1996
Women's Tennis	Ndali Ijomah	1,774	2000
Men's Track & Field	Brad Perry	1,589	2001
Swimming	Megan Sampson	1,410	2003
Men's Tennis	Jacek Wolicki	1,374	2002
Men's Gymnastics	Josh Raslie	1,267	2002

Performance Index combines points from 10, 40, VJ, and Pro Agility Run.

doing a leg press could never achieve a 2.0 grade for the lift. By making the players accountable, they use the poundage they are asked to and do the major lifts more regularly. This system pointed out very quickly who was being excused by the trainers. This system requires that supervisors keep accurate records, but it could be done at most high schools.

This grading system really made a difference. Scott Frost ended the 17-week season with a 1.90 average grade. Defensive back Mike Brown, now with the Chicago Bears, had the highest score on the team with a 1.97 average. He missed getting a 2 on one lift all season. Ahman Green, the starting I-back, began the season scoring a 2 on each workout until he was injured in week two and went five weeks before getting back to a 2 grade. His injury restricted him from doing the major lifts, so he received a lower grade. At midseason he was back doing squats and hang cleans but with a light weight, and by the end of the season he was again scoring a 2 grade on every lift. He finished the season by taking the national championship away from Tennessee in the second half by rushing for 206 yards and two

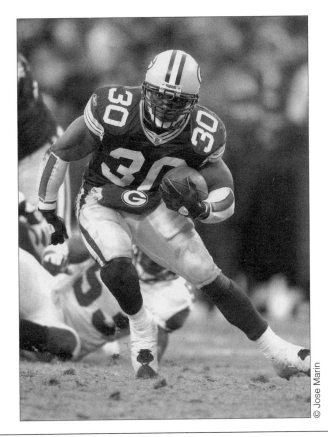

© Jose Marin

The grading system we implemented made a big difference in ensuring players were working at the proper intensity. It helped motivate players like Ahman Green, who has gone on to a successful career with the Green Bay Packers.

touchdowns. Ahman went on to a very productive career with the Seattle Seahawks and Green Bay Packers.

Some schools test then skip ahead and begin conditioning without the benefits of evaluation or goal setting. Part of the reason might be that these index points were not available the past 20 years. Now that they are, you can use them to motivate your athletes to set challenging goals. Using this information can help your program stand out from programs that don't take time to evaluate their athletes.

9

Goal Setting

Establishing goals is an essential element of any sports conditioning program. Without goals, a coach can't develop workouts that give direction and progressively increase intensity. It's unfortunate how many coaches have their athletes enter the weight room without first setting goals. Athletes make more progress if they know beforehand what they're trying to achieve. Set goals for yourself as a coach, for the team, and for each athlete.

Define Personal Missions

There's more to creating and attaining goals than saying, "I want to increase my squat 50 pounds and improve my 40-yard dash two-tenths of a second by the start of football season." Goal setting starts with the development of a strong, well-defined mission stating what you want to achieve. An athlete's personal mission might be to make the team or to make the all-state first team. It might be to earn a scholarship, play professionally, or make the Olympics. Most great athletes have a defined mission regarding what they want to accomplish. With their mission in mind, they set goals and determine how to achieve them. Athletes must make sacrifices and develop disciplined lifestyles to achieve the goals they set for themselves.

Coaches must develop a team philosophy and explain it to the team, encourage athletes to commit to developing to their fullest potential, and ask them to train hard without missing any workouts. Athletes must understand that you have a program that has been proven to work, but it will only work for them if they follow it religiously.

Have athletes write down their mission—what they expect of themselves, what they'll personally contribute. Have them sign it and keep it for motivation. Tell them they shouldn't share their personal mission with teammates until after they achieved it.

Set Goals With Your Athletes

Athletes should have most of the input when setting goals because this makes them more dedicated to achieve them. The role of the coach is to keep them from setting goals that are too high or too low. Point out their strengths and their weaknesses. Let your players know how dedicated to their workouts they will need to be to achieve their goals.

Goals should reflect the conclusions drawn from the evaluation of testing data. Tell athletes to focus on and set higher goals for areas in which they need the most improvement. You've heard the saying, "A chain is only as strong as its weakest link." As the weak link is improved, other components also improve.

When helping athletes set goals, keep in mind that they'll make more progress in their first year of a program than in succeeding years. As they get closer to reaching their potential, improvement will be more difficult. Sometimes there might be no improvement in a particular area. Help your athletes stay positive. Encourage them not to give up. Sometimes a step back in progress occurs because they're working too hard and not giving their bodies a chance to recover.

Keep good records that include testing information and all goals that have been set. Make sure all the information is dated.

Set Long- and Short-Range Goals

An athlete's long-range goal should be what he or she wants to achieve for the year. For example, an athlete whose current squat is at 330 pounds might set a goal to squat 380 pounds by the start of the next regular season.

Once long-range goals have been determined, short-range goals should then be set for each conditioning period during the year. Let's look at some examples of short-range goals for different periods. Because the emphasis of the 8-week postseason is to build a base, goals should not be set too high for this period. A 15-pound weight increase on the squat (for a total of 345 pounds) over the 8 weeks sounds about right. During the 12-week off-season, the objective is to gain strength. An appropriate goal for this period would be an increase of another 25 pounds (which would put him at 370 for the squat). For the 12-week preseason, he might set a goal to put on 10 more pounds on his squat, which would achieve his long-range goal of 380 pounds set before the start of the season.

Be flexible and allow adjustments in the goal-setting process. Goals aren't set in concrete. Athletes might reach their long-range goals sooner than expected and need to make new ones.

Nebraska strength coaches use the new Husker Power Strength Disk to generate lifting workouts each week. The strength disk allows coaches to increase poundage in a consistent manner based on the athletes' short-range goals. (You can purchase the disk at www.huskerpower.com.) A lifting workout is then printed out showing exactly how much weight to lift on a day-to-day, week-to-week basis. Athletes can then go into the weight room knowing exactly how much they must lift to keep on schedule and realize their goal. Without this type of program, many athletes enter the weight room excited at the prospect of achieving their goals early—then they progress at a rate that causes overtraining and premature peaking.

Set Challenging But Realistic Goals

If athletes' goals aren't realistic, the whole system breaks down. Athletes get discouraged and lose motivation to work their hardest. If athletes aren't motivated to reach their goals, they won't reach them. On the other hand, goals shouldn't be so easily attainable that they aren't challenging for athletes to achieve. This also results in low motivation. Athletes think, *I can reach this goal with no problem—why work on it now?*

To help athletes set goals that are challenging yet realistic it's best to compare their current data with their past testing results. Use the athlete's master profile, which includes all of his or her test scores, to see what kind of progress has been made in the past.

Once goals are achieved, help your athletes evaluate their progress and set new goals. Don't let them get too satisfied with themselves. There's always room for more improvement. Once they become satisfied, their work habits deteriorate, and they actually decline in their physical abilities. This often occurs when an athlete finally attains status as a first-stringer—he or she feels there's nothing left to achieve. Keep your starters motivated by having them continually set new goals.

No matter how little talent some athletes might have, they can still become successful members of your program. I have seen average athletes become All-Americans through hard work and high personal motivation. These are the kind of athletes you want in your program—those who won't quit until their goals are accomplished. No matter how many roadblocks or obstacles are put in their way, they keep going until their goal is reached. Their desire is so great that they're motivated to put in the long hours of training and practice, and to make the sacrifices necessary to succeed. Until then, they're not satisfied or happy. No reward is greater than an athlete's own personal happiness. They achieve happiness when they reach their goal. It's amazing how the simple feeling of happiness motivates people to work harder and achieve even greater goals.

Each of an athlete's lifting sessions and running workouts should be a stepping stone toward reaching his or her goal and, by extension, personal satisfaction and happiness. You can help your athletes by telling them what training needs to be done and how often to do it, but they must supply the rest. Their enthusiasm toward their workouts is very important. Enthusiasm can't be faked day after day, week after week. The workouts will become too long and too hard. They must have the desire, determination, and dedication to carry them to their goals. There are no shortcuts in the world of athletics—only goals to be set and reached. Athletes should feel guilty if they haven't done everything in their power to reach their full potential in life. Everyone likes to win, but not everyone will prepare to win. They can't always beat their opponents in talent, but if they use their will power, they can beat them in conditioning. How can you help? By staying positive and helping them stay positive. Don't ever let your athletes get down on themselves unless it's because of a lack of effort. Keep them focused on taking the steps toward achieving their goals. Celebrate their small successes along the way.

Goals aren't limited to athletes. Staff needs to set goals as well. Jeff Mangold was a student assistant with a goal of becoming a strength coach for a Major League baseball team. He made tremendous sacrifices to volunteer at Nebraska, and as money ran short, I let him drive the Husker Power van to help him stay afloat. Jeff was eventually hired by the University of Florida. During spring training, he was noticed by the New York Yankees. He reached his goal of becoming strength coach for the Yankees and helped them win three World Series titles in a row. He no longer worries about having a vehicle to drive.

The Husker Power program's principles give direction to the goal-setting process and provide a means for athletes to achieve the goals they have set. The performance staff makes many sacrifices of their time. They provide an edge with their research, but it's the athletes themselves who provide the Nebraska work ethic—which remains a mystery to visiting coaches trying to copy our program. Many observers think Nebraska is loaded with talent, but on closer inspection they find the real reason for success lies in the walk-on program. Hundreds of athletes in a variety of sports have come to Nebraska to develop physically. Compared to Texas, Oklahoma, and Colorado, Nebraska isn't known for recruiting a lot of talent. In the Big 12, recruiting classes usually favor the other schools. Coach Solich says, "Our recruiting classes might not be ranked number 1, but we go about things in our own way. We study films hard and make sure we're comfortable with players coming here to play for Nebraska." The 2002 figures showed 39 Huskers in the NFL. Colorado was next with

One quality that can make or break the success of an athletic program is the work ethic of the athletes. Coaches visiting the Nebraska campus are often amazed at how hard our athletes work. The visiting coaches always mention the intensity of the Nebraska workouts and the focus of the Nebraska athletes on doing the drills correctly.

The image of a successful athlete is one who works hard and does the job right. Successful athletes work hard because they want to but also because they are given the proper amount of rest. Several Nebraska athletes have had four-year careers without missing a single workout. The entire football team has gone through the six-week winter program (lifting four days per week and running four days per week) without one missed workout. The 1999 football team had 147 players in Lincoln doing their summer strength and conditioning. Every female basketball player and every female volleyball player also stayed in Lincoln all summer to train. The work ethic of Nebraska athletes is very impressive, and it brings results. In six weeks during winter conditioning, the 2000 football team gained 1,120 pounds of lean body mass.

37, followed by Texas A&M with 35, Kansas State with 27, Texas with 25, and Kansas and Oklahoma with 16 each.

Gil Brandt, who served as the director of player personnel for the Dallas Cowboys for 30 years and now writes a column for NFL.com says, "Nebraska does a good job of developing the players they have." He praised Nebraska's top-flight facilities, the academic support program, and the strength-conditioning program for preparing Nebraska's 30 first-round NFL draft picks.

Performance Pyramid

The symbol of Nebraska's performance program is a pyramid, which appears on the Performance Index and Strength Index T-shirts. The symbol is also on the food trays at the Performance Buffet. Over the years, Nebraska's Performance Team has worked to create a pyramid that ties in everything we're trying to achieve in our training process. We decided to use a pyramid shape to show how each block signifies a different component of training. Character is at the foundation because it creates the greatest changes, which in turn affects everything above it. As athletes develop character, they become more consistent in their conditioning habits. Better conditioning leads to greater athletic ability, which improves practice skills. Ultimately, these skills improve perfor-

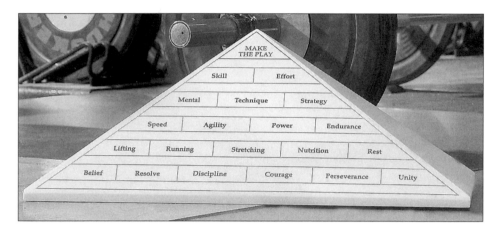

Figure 9.1   Nebraska's Performance Pyramid

mance potential. A white marble Performance Pyramid (see figure 9.1) is on display in Nebraska's strength complex to remind our athletes of these training components. A smaller version is given annually each spring to the male and female Husker Power Athlete of the Year.

Character

The character level of the pyramid consists of six components: belief, resolve, discipline, courage, perseverance, and unity. There are other components of character, but Tom Osborne stressed these six in his meetings with the Nebraska football players, and they make up the foundation of the Performance Pyramid. We ask, *Would your behavior be the same if you knew someone was watching you?* These components of the pyramid involve what people would do if they thought they'd never be found out. Coach Osborne wanted his athletes to develop a personal code of conduct based on their values and with a solid foundation leading to success in life beyond the athletic field.

Belief. To have great success, athletes need to have faith in the head coach of their sport. They also need to have faith in the strength and conditioning program and the people running it. If athletes don't believe in the plan, they won't be motivated to put in the effort required for the workouts. John Cook, Nebraska's volleyball coach, believes that his team is the most physical team on the court. He has never taken the court when he felt the other team was more physical than his athletes. Mike Arthur has done a lot of research over the years that has led to 10 principles presented in this book (see chapter 4). These principles have made our strength program more efficient, giving us an edge over opponents. As coaches and athletes hear about the principles and see the progress we've made, their belief in our program becomes even stronger.

Resolve. Resolve is a fixed purpose of mind to focus actions on the accomplishment of a specific goal. Athletes show resolve by developing a mission for what they want to achieve and then conducting themselves in a manner that completes the mission. If everyone focused on what they were supposed to do each day, championships would take care of themselves. Successful teams are those on which each member has the resolve to stay within a systematic approach while working toward a goal. Resolve is a lot like commitment. Steve Lindquist, an offensive guard for the Huskers, was born with one hand with no fingers. He resolved not to let this stand in his way as a Husker football player, refusing special treatment of any kind. When other players did hang cleans, he refused to be excused from the lift, requesting that I tape his hand to the bar. He had resolved to succeed despite any impedances, and he did.

Discipline. Discipline means following through on your resolve. It means doing the right thing at the right time. The structure of athletics—coming to practice on time, lifting weights on a regular schedule, running in the heat of summer—forces most young athletes to develop self-discipline,

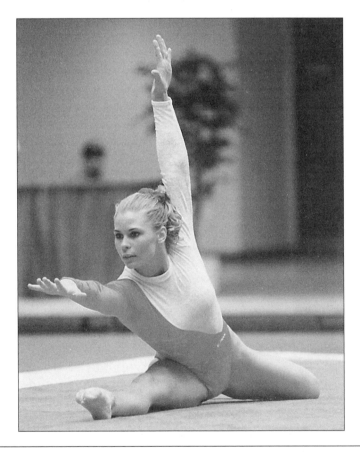

Successful athletes know it takes discipline to stay on the path to success.

which carries over to other parts of their life as well. Although they spend more time training than most other athletes, cross country runners and gymnasts always seem to have the best grades in school. Their success depends on a disciplined training schedule that allows time for study. Athletes need to decide if they'll give up activities that are counterproductive to athletic success. Discipline is a matter of replacing bad habits with good habits. At Nebraska, a sign on the exit door of the strength complex reads, "Your work habits determine your future!"

Courage. Courage is an important part of character. Because of fear, some athletes don't deal with their problems until it's too late, when the solution is very costly or out of their control. The best way to deal with fear is to face the problem head-on with courage. Courage enables a person to conquer fear. Each time a problem is met head-on and defeated, courage is strengthened. Sometimes it helps to view a problem within a worst-case scenario—if you can cope with and handle the worst you can imagine, anything less serious is a plus.

Doing what's right and not giving in to the popular view of others takes courage. It took some courage for quarterback Eric Crouch to stand before the media in New York City and accept the Heisman trophy in 2001, but it took much more courage for him to walk away from the NFL because he didn't feel right playing receiver. His decision had nothing to do with the NFL's money. He gave back the $395,000 bonus, thanked the NFL coaches, and walked away. He could have made $225,000 to stay on the payroll as an injured receiver, but Eric had the courage to do what he thought was the right thing for him regardless of what others thought of him. Some people called him a quitter and were disappointed in him. But many more were disappointed *for* him because he was never given the chance to show he could play his position in the pros. One thing is certain—Eric is a man with exceptional courage.

Perseverance. Perseverance means continuing to believe in yourself when facing adversity. You must be persistent and determined to reach your goals. If you continue to work hard and do things right, you'll get there. With ordinary talent and extraordinary perseverance, all things are possible. Matt Shaw was a walk-on football player for Nebraska who we really didn't expect to make the team. But he trained hard at practice and lifted weights with tremendous intensity. He was so far down the depth chart that he wasn't expected to ever play in a game. His perseverance kept him focused on his goal, and he never got discouraged. The many hours spent on the scout team running the opponents' plays against the top units never got him down. During his first years, he never got into games. But as a senior he was one of five players nominated for the Lifter of the Year award by his teammates. Matt came to me and said he didn't feel he deserved the honor. He wanted his name removed from the ballot. In my entire career I've never had an athlete who was so humble. Matt continued to train hard and practice with a passion, but he fell short of his goal as a receiver. He finished his career without ever catching a pass in a game. Matt shifted his perseverance to preparing for his medical degree, and now he is Dr. Matt Shaw. It's not always talent but perseverance that wins the race.

In the weight room, athletes reach training plateaus, and further progress seems impossible. Don't let them become discouraged. Setbacks are normal and necessary for progress. There are no short cuts. Help your athletes to take one step at a time and keep progressing until they reach their goal.

Kevin Steele, former Nebraska assistant, was head football coach at Baylor when he won his first Big-12 conference game against Kansas 35–32 by scoring 11 points in the final three minutes of the 2002 game. Baylor had 29 straight conference losses, the nation's record, before the win. Coach Steele told his players, "Don't ever give up," and eventually their perseverance paid off.

Unity. Team unity is an important cornerstone of the performance pyramid. Each athlete plays a role in contributing to the overall success of the team. The role might be as a back-up, a scout team member, or a captain. Success depends on each person doing his or her part. Putting teammates first builds team unity. A team might get a great effort from one person, but the effort leads to nothing because it's not in sync with what the rest of the team is doing. Winning doesn't challenge team unity like losing does. When losing, a team can either fall apart or pull together in spite of adversity. Playing well under adversity is the true test of team unity.

Nebraska replaced men's basketball coach Danny Nee after the 1999 season. Danny was a good coach, a former Marine with strong discipline. He coached several underdog Nebraska teams to wins over national powerhouse Kansas. But somewhere along the line, he lost team unity. For one reason or another, some of his players didn't believe in how he was doing things. Once a few players lose belief in the head coach, team unity erodes. Individuals pull in different directions, and discipline becomes a problem. For Danny, things got so bad that one night just minutes before the start of the game, a couple of his players who were scheduled to start couldn't be found on the floor as the team was shooting warm-up shots. The coaches and managers scrambled around looking for them and found them at the concession stand buying hot dogs. Team unity is one of the cornerstones of the Performance Pyramid. A program can't survive without it.

Conditioning

The conditioning segment of the pyramid includes stretching, lifting, nutrition, and rest. The proper application of these components allows good athletes to make great contributions and allows great players to become superstars.

Warm-up. Static stretches during which athletes hold a position for 10 to 15 seconds improve flexibility, but what most athletes really need is to warm up prior to the activity. Drills that improve mobility or get the blood circulating are much better for warm-up than stretching. Nebraska uses certain warm-up drills before practice or running workouts and other warm-up drills before lifting workouts.

Lifting. The purpose of a strength-training program is to improve performance. This means developing lean body mass, explosive power, and speed. Athletes who strength train tend to have fewer injuries because they have stronger muscle attachments and increased bone density. When injuries do occur for athletes with a solid background in lifting, they usually aren't serious and tend to heal faster.

Nutrition. Having enough energy to work out and practice is a primary concern for all athletes. Often, a decrease in performance can be traced back to improper nutrition. What an athlete eats determines how energy is supplied to the body before workouts and practices. After the workout, there's a small window of opportunity to replace nutrients used in workouts to speed recovery. At Nebraska we make sure our athletes take advantage of this window.

Rest. The body can't recover between workouts without enough rest. Athletes need to cut back on outside activities that interfere with recovery. They should get at least eight hours of quality sleep. Rest also applies to the amount of time required between sets and repetitions in lifting and the required down time between drills in conditioning.

Athletic Ability

The athletic ability part of the pyramid is made up of a set of attributes that athletes use in their sport. Most sports require speed, agility, power, and anaerobic endurance.

Speed. Speed involves getting from point A to point B as quickly as possible. Fast runners don't extend their legs any faster or have any quicker foot strikes than slower runners. What makes a difference is the amount of force applied against the ground. This is why athletes can become faster as they become stronger and bigger.

Agility. Regardless of the sport, being able to change directions and accelerate is a primary aspect. Quarterback Tommie Frazier didn't have great speed, but his amazing agility helped him to finish second in the Heisman trophy balloting in 1995. In a game against West Virginia, he changed directions six times in one play on his way to the end zone.

Power. Power is the rate at which work is accomplished. It involves how much strength can be expressed within a set amount of time. The greatest power is developed between 30 and 50 percent of maximum strength. To help your athletes become more powerful, include explosive lifts in your lifting program. Note that strength is related to power, but it's not the same thing. Strength has little to do with time, whereas power depends on time.

Endurance. Endurance involves maintaining maximum performance throughout an activity or contest. Athletes build endurance through interval training, which develops the ability to recover completely within a specified rest interval so that maximum intensity is possible for each work interval. Most power sports require interval training, not continuous training, to replace needed energy.

Practice

This level of the Performance Pyramid focuses on proper execution of what has been practiced. Practice consists of mental aspects, fundamentals, and strategies.

Mental aspects. Athletes should take the field or court with confidence that they have prepared well. Confidence comes from knowing assignments and being in better shape than opponents. Mental training also helps because the subconscious doesn't distinguish between what is vividly imagined and what is real.

Technique. Good technique is the medium through which power is expressed. When athletes are weak or injured, they can't express good technique because they don't have the required power.

Strategies. Game plans, or strategies, are devised by coaches to take best advantage of a team's strengths in light of an opponent's weaknesses.

Game

How a person plays in a game situation depends on factors that can't be measured with a stopwatch or tape measure. Some athletes can perform, whereas others struggle. Nebraska coaches look for high levels of both skill and effort in their athletes. Skill involves ability; effort involves strength of will.

Skill. Body control, hand–eye coordination, concentration, timing, and reaction are some of the attributes athletes are born with that can't always be coached. Some people lack the genetic ability to execute, whereas others are natural athletes.

Effort. Effort involves giving an intense attempt each time. It involves never giving up until a competition is over. Effort is a thread running throughout the Performance Pyramid. It takes effort to improve character, it takes effort to practice hard, and it takes effort to improve performance.

Performance

Athletes need to "make the play" when called on. An athlete's ability to perform depends on a combination of character, conditioning, athletic

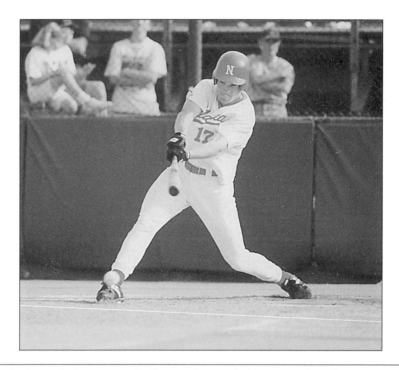

The fastest way to become a better performer is to set goals to increase strength and power.

ability, practice habits, skill level, and effort. The fastest way to become a better performer in most sports is to set goals to increase strength and power.

"Want To" Versus "Have To"

In 1990, the wheels fell off and Nebraska couldn't figure out what happened to the football program. We lost to Colorado 27–12 (the Buffs went on to win half a national championship that year). We lost to Oklahoma 45–10. We lost to Georgia Tech 45–21 (Georgia Tech won the other half of the championship that year). At the end of the year, we were 9–3. That doesn't sound too bad for most teams, but finishing out of the top 10 for the first time in 20 years caused some serious finger pointing.

We seemed to have enough talent on the team, but too many players had bad attitudes, and punishing them didn't help. Many players had little respect and little self-discipline. For years I had a punishment system in place for players who missed lifting. I had players do grass drills or stadium steps or up-and-downs.

Some players never missed a workout. I-Back Jeff Smith, for example, had no absences over his entire career. But in 1990 an average of 40 players missed their lifting workout each day. We had a senior with 140 absences from lifting over his career. Some players reached the point where they were choosing the punishment rather than doing the workout. Somehow, players had forgotten what had made the program successful for 20 years.

On January 17, 1991, I decided to hold a meeting to address these issues. The meeting room was noisy; players were talking and not paying attention as Dennis LeBlanc, director of academic services, made his announcements. It was normal for Dennis to speak first, but this time the players didn't quiet down, and many didn't pay attention. When Dennis was finished, I went to the front of the auditorium and held up a paperweight shaped like a national championship ring. I didn't say anything but just held up the ring. As the players began noticing I wasn't talking, the room got very quiet. In fact, it got so quiet it was scary. Once I had the players' attention, I said, "This is what a national championship ring looks like. I have a plan to help you earn such a ring, but I need your help. We need to make some changes, and the changes will have to come from you." I explained that all athletic teams have three groups of players. I then drew a circle on the bulletin board with three segments, like a pie chart.

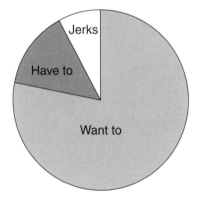

Three groups on a team.

The "want to" group on a team usually has no absences; these players are on the team because they want to be there, and they always do a good job. The "have to" guys are on the team because someone told them to be. They don't always want to be there, but they know they have to stay on the team for one reason or another. Players in the "have to" group can do everything right, just like the "want to" guys, but "have to" players can also easily slip into the third segment of the pie. It's because of the "have to" group that we developed a system at Nebraska in which each lifting session is graded. It's not enough to just attend and do a workout. The work must be *quality* work. Attendance alone is not enough.

For lack of a better name, I called the third group "jerks." Players in this group don't go to class regularly, they don't work out regularly, and they jerk around in all phases of their life. They really don't belong on the team and can seriously damage the team's direction. Jerks need to be eliminated from the program.

I explained to the group of 200 players that they were averaging 40 absences a day in their lifting workouts. I said, "This is not acceptable," and I offered a two-step plan. "Step one is to eliminate the jerks in this program, and we're going to start that right now. From this day forward there will be no more punishment for missing lifting or running. Starting tomorrow you come because you want to. If you choose not to come, don't come back. If you miss, you're done."

Then I pointed out that players would be allowed one absence as a warning during the six-week program, but if they missed more than once they would be off the team. I twice asked for any player who did not want to be part of the program to leave. When no one left the room, I went back to the board and changed the drawing by erasing the "jerk" segment. Now only two categories remained, and step one was completed.

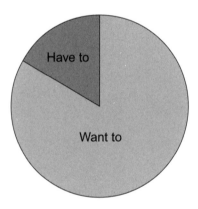

"Want to" and "have to" groups remain.

As I pointed to the two-group chart, I said, "Okay, the second step in getting you all championship rings is to motivate the 'have to' guys to be 'want to' guys." I then spent quite a bit of time explaining that inside each athlete are two little voices that talk to them several times a day. These voices debate about what's right and wrong. I explained to them that when the alarm went off in the morning, the "want to" part of them was ready to hop up and go. "This part of you never gives up; this part of you takes pride, has a positive attitude, and is committed to a goal or mission. This part of you does not miss workouts; this is the part of you that appears in your visions. You can call this part 'Will Power,' and he's in every one of you." I further explained that Will Power comes from within. "He has to come from you; you can use him to control your actions." Then I asked the players to do everything requested of them for the next six weeks. I wouldn't yell at them or punish them; these are negatives and don't work. The only way for the program to work was for them to want to do things right. I then asked them to stand up if they were willing to commit to doing the program right. It was a pretty scary feeling to have 200 players standing in close quarters, so motivated they could run through a wall. At that point I returned to the board and erased the "have to" piece of the pie chart, leaving us with 100 percent "want to" athletes—the way it should be.

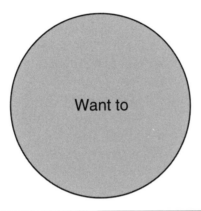

100 percent "want to" athletes.

My staff then handed out red practice jerseys to everyone in the room, and I asked the players to wear their jerseys each day as a reminder of their mission. Over the next six weeks if someone showed up to work out without his red jersey, he was sent back to the locker room to get it. We had 200 players lifting four sessions a week and running four sessions a week. Players made it to 6,500 workouts with only 7 individual absences before we lost our starting middle guard because he missed his second workout. A few days later, we lost our starting I-Back, the Big Eight's leading rusher the year before. Coach Osborne wanted to know what was going on. He had recruited these players, was in their homes, and knew their families, and now because they had missed two workouts in the off-season they were off the team. I reminded Coach Osborne that all the players had committed and agreed to this plan. They had the choice each day of being on the team or not. Fortunately, Coach Osborne supported the discipline. He lost two players, but he got back a football team with a tremendous attitude. He had observed the turn-around attitude and knew how hard the players were working to do things right. No one else missed a workout.

In March 1991, the day before the six-week winter program was over, I got the team together and told them, "Testing at the conclusion of the six-week winter conditioning program usually produces 15 to 18 new school records each year. I expect 50 school records to be broken tomorrow!" I knew they had worked harder than they ever had before, with almost no misses. I felt confident they had made great progress. I wanted to plant a seed of confidence in their minds. The next day, they broke 78 school records. No one had ever seen such an improvement. The players were relentless in their workouts. The policy put in place that winter was a drastic step that worked. The freshmen in that meeting on January 17, 1991, continued to work hard throughout their careers. In 1994, their senior year, they won a national championship ring after winning four straight Big Eight championships.

The starting offensive linemen from that 1994 national championship team were considered the best in Nebraska history and maybe in the entire nation. Four of the five were freshmen in that turn-around meeting on January 17, 1991.

The bottom line in the strength and conditioning field is the mind controls the body. If the athletes don't want to work hard and improve, they won't. Somehow you need to sell them that you can help them if they follow your program. If you choose to use the recommended program, you can tell them this program is guaranteed to improve their performance.

10

Program Design

A progressive and methodical application of overload in an athlete's program over time provides the stimulus and the needed recovery to produce the best results. This means drills and exercises must be combined systematically to improve the strength, conditioning, speed, and agility necessary to play at a championship level. Exercises and drills must be organized into a plan on a yearly basis to peak athletes as they go into the season. To help you develop your annual plan, study the "Big Picture" as shown in tables 10.1 through 10.3.

Big Picture

The first step in program design is to look at a calendar and determine which months your athletes should train. Depending on the sport, divide the year into four seasons in a building-block format. Each season lays the foundation for the next, more intense, season.

In increments of 12-week cycles, count backward from where the season starts. Each cycle contains three 4-week phases. (The postseason does not allow for 12 weeks, so only the base and development phases are included in the table.) During the off-season and preseason, strength levels are determined at the *end* of each 4-week phase during the workout for both explosive lifts and strength lifts. Note that the number of repetitions used to measure strength levels corresponds to the number of reps that have been done during the 4-week training period. For example, the fall-sport Big Picture calls for strength-level checks in weeks 13, 17, 21, 26, and 30 and an official strength

FALL SPORT

Table 10.1   Fall Sport

			Phase		Explosive	Strength	Conditioning
Postseason	January	1	Base		3 × 5	3 × 10	Active rest
		2	Base		3 × 5	3 × 10	Active rest
		3	Base	Unload	3 × 5	3 × 10	Active rest
		4	Base		3 × 5	3 × 10	Active rest
	February	5	Development		3 × 3	3 × 5	Active rest
		6	Development		3 × 3	3 × 5	Active rest
		7	Development	Unload	3 × 3	3 × 5	Active rest
		8	Development		3 × 3	3 × 5	Active rest
Off-season	March	9	Active rest				Active rest
		10	Base		3 × 5	3 × 10	Active rest
		11	Base		3 × 5	3 × 10	Active rest
		12	Base	Unload	3 × 5	3 × 10	Active rest
		13	Base	Strength level	5-6 reps	10 reps	Active rest
	April	14	Development		3 × 3	3 × 5	Active rest
		15	Development		3 × 3	3 × 5	Active rest
		16	Development	Unload	3 × 3	3 × 5	Active rest
		17	Development	Strength level	3-4 reps	3-5 reps	Active rest
	May	18	Peak		4/3/2	10,8,6,4,3,2	Active rest
		19	Peak		4/3/2	10,8,6,4,3,2	Active rest
		20	Peak	Unload	4/3/2	10,8,6,4,3,2	Active rest
		21	Peak	Strength level	1-2 reps	1-3 reps	Active rest
Preseason	June	22	Active rest				Active rest
		23	Base	New level	3 × 5	3 × 10	Active rest
		24	Base		3 × 5	3 × 10	Active rest
		25	Base	Unload	3 × 5	3 × 10	Active rest
		26	Base	Strength level	5-6 reps	10 reps	Active rest

			Phase		Explosive	Strength	Conditioning
		27	Development		3 × 3	3 × 5	Speed
		28	Development		3 × 3	3 × 5	Speed
	July	29	Development	Unload	3 × 3	3 × 5	Speed
		30	Development	Strength level	3-4 reps	3-5 reps	Speed
		31	Peak		4/3/2	10,8.6,4,3,2	Speed & agility
		32	Peak		4/3/2	10,8.6,4,3,2	Speed & agility
	August	33	Peak	Unload	4/3/2	10,8.6,4,3,2	Speed & agility
		34	Peak	Test	1-2 reps	1-3 reps	Speed & agility
		35	Active rest				Active rest
In-Season		36	Maintenance		3 × 5	3 × 5	Football
		37	Maintenance		3 × 5	3 × 5	Football
	September	38	Maintenance	Unload	3 × 5	3 × 5	Football
		39	Maintenance		3 × 5	3 × 5	Football
		40	Maintenance		3 × 5	3 × 5	Football
		41	Maintenance		3 × 5	3 × 5	Football
	October	42	Maintenance	Unload	3 × 5	3 × 5	Football
		43	Maintenance		3 × 5	3 × 5	Football
		44	Maintenance		3 × 5	3 × 5	Football
		45	Maintenance		3 × 5	3 × 5	Football
	November	46	Maintenance	Unload	3 × 5	3 × 5	Football
		47	Maintenance		3 × 5	3 × 5	Football
		48	Maintenance		3 × 5	3 × 5	Football
		49	Maintenance	Unload	3 × 5	3 × 5	Football
	December	50	Active rest				Active rest
		51	Active rest				Active rest
		52	Active rest				Active rest

WINTER SPORT

			Phase		Explosive	Strength	Conditioning
In-season	January	1	Maintenance		3 × 5	3 × 5	Basketball
		2	Maintenance	Unload	3 × 5	3 × 5	Basketball
		3	Maintenance		3 × 5	3 × 5	Basketball
		4	Maintenance		3 × 5	3 × 5	Basketball
		5	Maintenance		3 × 5	3 × 5	Basketball
	February	6	Maintenance	Unload	3 × 5	3 × 5	Basketball
		7	Maintenance		3 × 5	3 × 5	Basketball
		8	Maintenance		3 × 5	3 × 5	Basketball
		9	Maintenance	Unload	3 × 5	3 × 5	Basketball
Postseason	March	10	Active rest				Active rest
		11	Active rest				Active rest
		12	Active rest				Active rest
		13	Active rest				Active rest
		14	Active rest				Active rest
	April	15	Base		3 × 5	3 × 10	Active rest
		16	Base		3 × 5	3 × 10	Active rest
		17	Base	Unload	3 × 5	3 × 10	Active rest
		18	Base		3 × 5	3 × 10	Active rest
	May	19	Development		3 × 3	3 × 5	Active rest
		20	Development		3 × 3	3 × 5	Active rest
		21	Development	Unload	3 × 3	3 × 5	Active rest
		22	Development		3 × 3	3 × 5	Active rest
		23	Active rest				Active rest
Off-season	June	24	Base		3 × 5	3 × 10	Active rest
		25	Base		3 × 5	3 × 10	Active rest
		26	Base	Unload	3 × 5	3 × 10	Active rest
		27	Base	Strength level	5-6 reps	10 reps	Active rest

Table 10.2 Winter Sport

			Phase		Explosive	Strength	Conditioning
Preseason	July	28	Development		3 × 3	3 × 5	Active rest
		29	Development		3 × 3	3 × 5	Active rest
		30	Development	Unload	3 × 3	3 × 5	Active rest
		31	Development	Strength level	3-4 reps	3-5 reps	Active rest
	August	32	Peak		4/3/2	10,8,6,4,3,2	Active rest
		33	Peak		4/3/2	10,8,6,4,3,2	Active rest
		34	Peak	Unload	4/3/2	10,8,6,4,3,2	Active rest
		35	Peak	Strength level	1-2 reps	1-3 reps	Active rest
		36	Active rest				Active rest
	September	37	Base	New level	3 × 5	3 × 10	Active rest
		38	Base		3 × 5	3 × 10	Active rest
		39	Base	Unload	3 × 5	3 × 10	Active rest
		40	Base	Strength level	5-6 reps	10 reps	Active rest
	October	41	Development		3 × 3	3 × 5	Speed
		42	Development		3 × 3	3 × 5	Speed
		43	Development	Unload	3 × 3	3 × 5	Speed
		44	Development	Strength level	3-4 reps	3-5 reps	Speed
	November	45	Peak		4/3/2	10,8,6,4,3,2	Speed & agility
		46	Peak		4/3/2	10,8,6,4,3,2	Speed & agility
		47	Peak	Unload	4/3/2	10,8,6,4,3,2	Speed & agility
		48	Peak	Test	1-2 reps	1-3 reps	Speed & agility
In-season	December	49	Active rest				Active rest
		50	Maintenance		3 × 5	3 × 5	Basketball
		51	Maintenance		3 × 5	3 × 5	Basketball
		52	Maintenance	Unload	3 × 5	3 × 5	Basketball

SPRING SPORT

Table 10.3　Spring Sport

			Phase		Explosive	Strength	Conditioning
Preseason	**January**	1	Development		3 × 3	3 × 5	Speed
		2	Development		3 × 3	3 × 5	Speed
		3	Development	Unload	3 × 3	3 × 5	Speed
		4	Development	Strength level	3-4 reps	3-5 reps	Speed
	February	5	Peak		4/3/2	10,8,6,4,3,2	Speed & agility
		6	Peak		4/3/2	10,8,6,4,3,2	Speed & agility
		7	Peak	Unload	4/3/2	10,8,6,4,3,2	Speed & agility
		8	Peak	Test	1-2 reps	1-3 reps	Speed & agility
		9	Active rest				Active rest
In-season	**March**	10	Maintenance		3 × 5	3 × 5	Track
		11	Maintenance	Unload	3 × 5	3 × 5	Track
		12	Maintenance		3 × 5	3 × 5	Track
		13	Maintenance		3 × 5	3 × 5	Track
	April	14	Maintenance		3 × 5	3 × 5	Track
		15	Maintenance	Unload	3 × 5	3 × 5	Track
		16	Maintenance		3 × 5	3 × 5	Track
		17	Maintenance		3 × 5	3 × 5	Track
	May	18	Maintenance		3 × 5	3 × 5	Track
		19	Maintenance	Unload	3 × 5	3 × 5	Track
		20	Maintenance		3 × 5	3 × 5	Track
		21	Maintenance		3 × 5	3 × 5	Track
		22	Maintenance	Unload	3 × 5	3 × 5	Track

			Phase		Explosive	Strength	Conditioning
Postseason	**June**	23	Active rest				Active rest
		24	Active rest				Active rest
		25	Active rest				Active rest
		26	Active rest				Active rest
	July	27	Base		3 × 5	3 × 10	Active rest
		28	Base		3 × 5	3 × 10	Active rest
		29	Base	Unload	3 × 5	3 × 10	Active rest
		30	Base		3 × 5	3 × 10	Active rest
	August	31	Development		3 × 3	3 × 5	Active rest
		32	Development		3 × 3	3 × 5	Active rest
		33	Development	Unload	3 × 3	3 × 5	Active rest
		34	Development		3 × 3	3 × 5	Active rest
		35	Active rest				Active rest
Off-season	**September**	36	Base		3 × 5	3 × 10	Active rest
		37	Base		3 × 5	3 × 10	Active rest
		38	Base	Unload	3 × 5	3 × 10	Active rest
		39	Base	Strength level	5-6 reps	10 reps	Active rest
	October	40	Development		3 × 3	3 × 5	Active rest
		41	Development		3 × 3	3 × 5	Active rest
		42	Development	Unload	3 × 3	3 × 5	Active rest
		43	Development	Strength level	3-4 reps	3-5 reps	Active rest
	November	44	Peak		4/3/2	10,8,6,4,3,2	Active rest
		45	Peak		4/3/2	10,8,6,4,3,2	Active rest
		46	Peak	Unload	4/3/2	10,8,6,4,3,2	Active rest
		47	Peak	Strength level	1-2 reps	1-3 reps	Active rest
Preseason	**December**	48	Active rest				Active rest
		49	Base		3 × 5	3 × 10	Active rest
		50	Base		3 × 5	3 × 10	Active rest
		51	Base	Unload	3 × 5	3 × 10	Active rest
		52	Base	Strength level	5-6 reps	10 reps	Active rest

test in week 34. The strength-level check is done during a workout to determine where the athlete is for that portion of the 12-week cycle. The check involves simply lifting as much weight as possible for the prescribed reps as outlined for the strength-level check in the Big Picture. A week of active rest is provided between cycles. Week 34 is a strength test done not in a workout session but with teammates watching and cheering.

Be specific with your objectives for each of the four training periods. Don't expect athletes to improve in all areas at the same time.

Postseason

This is a time to reflect, reevaluate, set goals, and build a foundation base of strength. It's also a time to recover and get away from structure. Immediately after the competitive season is over, athletes need rest. They need to recuperate physically and psychologically after a stressful season. If your athletes don't get some rest following the competitive season, they'll get stale and lose their enthusiasm to reach the intensity that's necessary for a conditioning response to occur. The most important time to take rest is right after the season. Encourage your athletes to use the active rest concept; tell them it's crucial to taking their physical development to higher levels. Sometimes athletes, wanting to show what hard workers they are, will train right through the active rest period. Doing so will diminish their ability to reach their long-range gains. Teach them to train smarter, not harder. Active rest is a time to have fun while being active enough to get a conditioning effect.

Choose conditioning activities that are enjoyable and that involve agility, reaction, and coordination. Basketball, racquetball, and tennis are excellent choices for the postseason. Control athletes' eating habits during active rest and have them work on developing great lifting technique. After the period of active rest, begin to focus on lifting technique, especially for the platform lifts.

Off-Season

The off-season program is similar to the postseason except it's more intense and includes all 12 weeks. The objective is to achieve maximum gains by building on the strength established in the postseason program. This is the time to get strong. Athletes can continue to participate in athletic activities, such as basketball or racquetball. Higher volume is done during the off-season, which means supplemental exercises are included during the base and development phases but are normally dropped during the peak and maintenance phases. The normal 4-week training period calls for "backing off" intensity for the 3rd week and a strength-level check during the 4th week. See figure 10.1.

The "backoff" (or "unload") phase can be achieved by reducing the percentage of weight used. Unloading also means doing two sets during supplemental exercises instead of three sets.

The Husker Power poundage chart (see Appendix, pages 307-312) is designed to make it very simple to choose poundages during a workout. To begin using the chart, refer to the following explanation as a guide.

The numbers at the very top of the chart represent workout routines used in the Husker Power recommended program. They include 3 × 10, 3 × 5, 3 × 3, 10/8/6/4/3/2, and 4/3/2. The column directly below each number contains the weight to be used for that set in the workout. The numbers in the far left column under "1RM" represent projected one-rep maximums for each exercise.

Recommended percentages

Week	Phase	Reps	Percentage
1	Base	3 X 10	65
2	Base	3 X 10	70
3	Unload	3 X 10	60
4	Test	10	75
5	Development	3 X 5	75
6	Development	3 X 5	80
7	Unload	3 X 5	70
8	Test	5	85

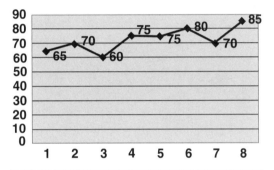

Figure 10.1   Recommended lifting percentages.

The horizontal column next to a given 1RM shows the required poundage for the workout. For example, if the workout calls for three sets of 10 reps, look down the 1RM column and find a workout that can be accomplished with proper technique. For instance, if the chosen 1RM is 200 pounds for three sets of 10, the three sets would be 130, 140, and 150 pounds (see table 10.4). If the sets and reps are completed with proper technique, the 1RM for that exercise is 200 lbs. If the poundages are easy, increase the 1RM the next workout. If the poundages are difficult and don't allow good technique, reduce the 1RM the next workout.

Preseason

Preseason is the period 12 weeks prior to the start of in-season practices. Your objective is to peak your athletes for the season. Drop assistance exercises and concentrate on the core or major exercises. Increase the intensity and lower the volume. Begin agility and speed drills as the season nears.

Table 10.4 Husker Power Poundage Chart

							3	3	3		5	5	5
1RM	10	10	10	10	8	6	4	3	2		4	3	2
190	125	135	140	95	115	135	150	160	170	140	150	160	170
195	125	135	145	95	115	135	155	165	175	145	155	165	175
200	130	140	150	100	120	140	160	170	180	150	160	170	180
205	135	145	155	100	125	145	165	175	185	155	165	175	185
210	135	145	155	105	125	145	170	180	190	155	170	180	190
215	140	150	160	105	130	150	170	180	195	160	170	180	195
220	145	155	165	110	130	155	175	185	200	165	175	185	200
225	145	155	170	110	135	155	180	190	200	170	180	190	200
230	150	160	170	115	140	160	185	195	205	170	185	195	205
235	150	165	175	115	140	165	190	200	210	175	190	200	210
240	155	170	180	120	145	170	190	205	215	180	190	205	215
245	160	170	185	120	145	170	195	210	220	185	195	210	220
250	160	175	185	125	150	175	200	210	225	185	200	210	225
255	165	180	190	125	155	180	205	215	230	190	205	215	230
260	170	180	195	130	155	180	210	220	235	195	210	220	235

In-Season

The objective for most programs during the in-season is to maintain strength levels acquired through the previous three training periods. However, for some sports, such as track and swimming, it can be wise to revisit the strength phase and peak phase during the season to bring about a peak toward the end of the season when the bigger meets are held. For football, do the "heavy day" workout earlier in the week because competition is at the end of the week. Maintaining strength levels during the season makes athletes less vulnerable to injuries and helps them recover if an injury does occur.

Multisport athletes in high school are always in a competitive season and never get the opportunity to advance through the other three training periods that make up the annual program. As a result, they never develop maximum strength and power. A program for the multisport athlete is shown in table 12.2 in chapter 12.

Specificity

Specificity relates to training with consideration of the particular athlete's sport season. The term refers to the method of training an athlete in a

What, No Running?

Zach Duval, a former strength coach for Nebraska, provided some post-test data that clearly shows athletes can improve speed, power, and agility without running a step.

Zach Duval did something I've always wanted to do. He proved that lifting with no running for six weeks will increase speed, agility, and power. I've always been involved with coaches that thought running was the most important component in the off-season. Zach trained high-school athletes in Colorado at a location in which he had no indoor fieldhouse to run in. He followed the Husker Power principles for six weeks in his lifting program and did no running. His pretest and post-test data show how his athletes were able to improve in all performance tests from lifting. I hope this kind of success gives other coaches confidence to conduct *lifting only* off-season programs when running is not possible. In fact, there should a period in the off-season during which the focus is getting strong without any running to interfere with recovery. Once the strength is gained, it's relatively easy to maintain it, so it's okay to begin running again. But when athletes adhere to programs that involve running all the time, they never get full strength benefits. The chart clearly shows an improvement for both male and female in every performance category, which proves that lifting weights and increasing force against the ground improves speed, agility, and power.

Data on High School Athletes

36 males lifting with no running—6 weeks pre/post averages

	10	40	Pro agility	VJ	Performance Index
Date: 11/13/2002	2.08	5.9	5.22	16.18	581.57
Date: 12/20/2002	1.86	5.7	5.06	20.9	770.54
Improvement	0.22	0.2	0.16	4.72	188.97

25 females lifting with no running—6 weeks pre/post averages

	10	40	Pro agility	VJ	Performance Index
Date: 1/11/2003	2.11	6.17	5.34	15.7	805
Date: 2/23/2003	1.89	5.82	4.97	20.33	1284
Improvement	0.22	0.35	0.37	4.63	479

© Zachary P. Duvall, The Explosive Edge

specific manner to produce a specific adaptation or training outcome. As an athlete progresses through the training periods, all forms of training should progress in an organized manner from general to sport specific. Specificity also ensures that muscles involved in selected exercises are those that the sport relies on and that the loads assigned are sufficient to challenge the athlete to become stronger and faster.

Regardless of the type of training program you choose, several principles always apply. Study the 10 principles in chapter 4 and make sure the exercises that are selected fit these principles. Principles for women should be the same as for men. The program should consist of multiple-joint exercises that are ground based and done explosively. The program should be designed to improve performance, not appearance.

Some exercises, such as the hang clean and power press, duplicate the contraction velocities used during jumping actions. More power is developed doing a hang clean, power press, or vertical jump than in doing a one-repetition maximum squat. The hang clean, power press, and vertical jump are true tests of power.

Both eccentric contractions (stretching of a muscle) and concentric contractions (shortening of a muscle) occur when executing many sport skills that require a maximum rate of force development. An eccentric contraction followed by a concentric contraction is known as the "stretch shortening cycle." When the muscle is stretched, an elastic energy is built up in it. The muscle then fights to return to its normal resting length (think of stretching a rubber band). If the muscles shorten immediately after the stretch, greater force and power can be generated. When executing a jump, the downward movement stretches the muscles and tendons of the hips, knees, and ankles. An elastic energy is built up in these muscles, and if the direction of the jump is reversed quickly, a greater force is generated, enabling the body to go higher.

Choose exercises based on the needs of the sport. The exercises should be performed in this order—large muscle group exercises first followed by small muscle groups.

More research needs to be done before coaches are going to buy into lifting programs with no running in the off-season. The recommended program calls for long periods of active rest which will be hard for some coaches to understand but if strength, power, muscle mass and speed improvement are goals, then take another look at the test results Zach Duval received. He now works in Omaha, Nebraska and is available to do clinics across the country. He can be reached by going to the huskerpower.com Web site and clicking on clinics.

11

Off-Season Programs

This chapter provides a recommended warm-up followed by a detailed explanation of explosive lifts. Coaches are then given three choices for slow movements, the traditional strength lifts, the push–pull circuit, or the metabolic circuit.

Warm-Up Drills

The lifting warm-up consists of two warm-up exercises. The snatch squat warm-up and hurdle drill warm-up are done prior to lifting before explosive day and strength day exercises. A separate warm-up is used for conditioning workouts.

Snatch Squat

The snatch squat warms up and stretches the hips, legs, and shoulders and helps develop total body stability and balance.

1. Place the bar on the racks at chest height.
2. Position hands on the bar slightly wider than shoulder-width apart.
3. Position the bar comfortably across the top of shoulders at the base of the neck.
4. Lift the bar out of the rack by extending the knees.
5. Step backward using as few steps as possible.
6. Position feet so they're parallel and toes are pointed out slightly.

7. The heels should be slightly wider than the hips.
8. Move hands to a snatch grip.
9. Press the bar overhead until arms are fully extended and squat down (figure 11.1).

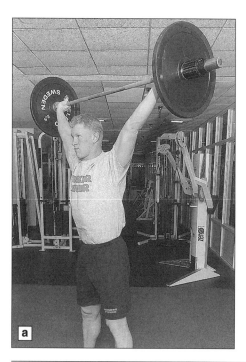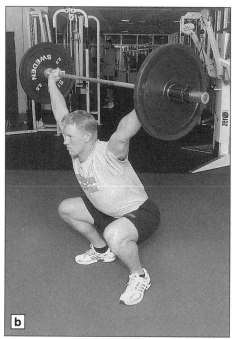

Figure 11.1 Snatch squat warm-up.

Key Points

- Press out hard on the bar during the entire movement.
- Keep the chest up and back straight during the entire movement.
- As you lower into the squat position, keep the bar positioned behind the head.

Hurdle Drill

This warm-up drill is done using a regulation track hurdle that can be adjusted in height according to an athlete's flexibility. This drill is for mobility and flexibility in the hip joints.

1. Stand perpendicular near one side of the hurdle.
2. Line up shoulders, hips, and feet in squared position.
3. Use slow, deliberate movements to glide under the hurdle and stand erect on the other side (figure 11.2).
4. Repeat going under the hurdle slowly with no jerky movements for a set of 10 repetitions.

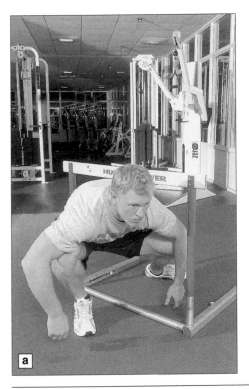
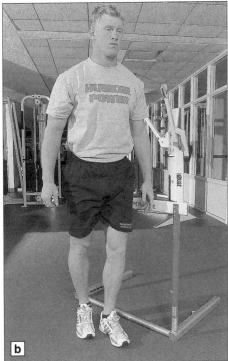

Figure 11.2   Hurdle drill warm-up.

Key Points
- Don't let your hands touch the ground or hurdle.
- Keep hips below the shoulders in the low squat position.
- Maintain a rhythmic stepping pattern under the hurdles.

Explosive Exercises

As the athletes progress from the four-week base phase to the four-week development phase, the exercise choice changes from rack clean to hang clean. Later, during the four-week peak phase, the lift is changed again to the power clean done from the floor. The program calls for another progression on explosive exercise number two. See the Explosive Day Program in table 11.1.

Rack clean, hang clean, and power clean

Standing front press, power press, and push jerk

Jammer extension

Pulling choice: pull-ups, standing low row, lat pull-down, or bent-over row

Biceps choice

The four-day recommended off-season program is divided into two days of explosive exercises and two days of strength exercises. See the recommended off-season explosive day program in tables 11.1–11.4.

The progress charts provide a space to record the poundage used and number of repetitions achieved as well as a space for the coach's initials. The charts identify the day of the week, name and number of exercise, number of recommended sets, and recommended repetitions for each week.

Table 11.1 Recommended Explosive Day Program

Exercise 1	Clean progression		
	Base	*1a. Rack clean (Master the shrug and clean catch before rack clean)	At the end of the base period, in the off-season and preseason, determine 1RM strength level as part of the workout for 5 to 6 reps
	Development	*1b. Hang clean	At the end of the development period, in the off-season and preseason, determine 1RM strength level as part of the workout for 3 to 4 reps
	Peak	*1c. Power clean	At the end of the peak period, in the off-season and preseason, determine 1RM strength level as part of the workout for 1 to 2 reps
Exercise 2	Press progression		
	Base	2a. Standing press	
	Development	2b. Power press	
	Peak	2c. Push jerk	
Exercise 3	3. Hammer jammer extension		
Exercise 4	**Pulling choice—4a. pull-ups, 4b. standing low row, 4c. lat pull-down, or 4d. bent-over row		
Exercise 5	5. Biceps choice		

*Test and determine strength levels on these major exercises.

**The pulling choice and biceps choice use three sets of 10 throughout the program.

Football athletes need to add a neck exercise—it's not explosive but can be done on explosive day.

Young athletes need to use a weight light enough to do at least 6 reps but not more than 15.

Table 11.2 Explosive Base

Monday	Week 1		Week 2		Week 3		Week 4	
Hurdle warm-up	2 × 5		2 × 5		2 × 5		2 × 5	
Snatch squat	2 × 5		2 × 5		2 × 5		2 × 5	
1a. Rack clean	3 × 5		3 × 5		3 × 5		3 × 5	
2a. Standing press	3 × 5		3 × 5		3 × 5		3 × 5	
3. Hammer jammer extension	3 × 5		3 × 5		3 × 5		3 × 5	
**4. Pulling choice	3 × 10		3 × 10		3 × 10		3 × 10	
5. Biceps choice	3 × 10		3 × 10		3 × 10		3 × 10	
Thursday				**Unload**				
Hurdle warm-up	2 × 5		2 × 5		2 × 5		2 × 5	
Snatch squat	2 × 5		2 × 5		2 × 5		2 × 5	
1a. Rack clean	3 × 5		3 × 5		3 × 5		3 × 5	
2a. Standing press	3 × 5		3 × 5		3 × 5		3 × 5	
3. Hammer jammer extension	3 × 5		3 × 5		3 × 5		3 × 5	
**4. Pulling choice	3 × 10		3 × 10		3 × 10		3 × 10	
5. Biceps choice	3 × 10		3 × 10		3 × 10		3 × 10	
Date	**Comments**						**INT**	
	**4a. pull-ups, 4b. standing low row, 4c. lat pull-down, or 4d. bent-over row							
	Football athletes need to add a neck exercise.							

Table 11.3 Explosive Development

Monday	Week 1		Week 2		Week 3		Week 4	
Hurdle warm-up	2 × 5		2 × 5		2 × 5		2 × 5	
Snatch squat	2 × 5		2 × 5		2 × 5		2 × 5	
1b. Hang clean	3 × 3		3 × 3		3 × 3		3 × 3	
2b. Power press	3 × 3		3 × 3		3 × 3		3 × 3	
3. Hammer jammer extension	3 × 3		3 × 3		3 × 3		3 × 3	
**4. Pulling choice	3 × 10		3 × 10		3 × 10		3 × 10	
5. Biceps choice	3 × 10		3 × 10		3 × 10		3 × 10	
Thursday	**Unload**							
Hurdle warm-up	2 × 5		2 × 5		2 × 5		2 × 5	
Snatch squat	2 × 5		2 × 5		2 × 5		2 × 5	
1b. Hang clean	3 × 3		3 × 3		3 × 3		3 × 3	
2b. Power press	3 × 3		3 × 3		3 × 3		3 × 3	
3. Hammer jammer extension	3 × 3		3 × 3		3 × 3		3 × 3	
**4. Pulling choice	3 × 10		3 × 10		3 × 10		3 × 10	
5. Biceps choice	3 × 10		3 × 10		3 × 10		3 × 10	
Date	**Comments**							**INT**
	**4a. pull-ups, 4b. standing low row, 4c. lat pull-down, or 4d. bent-over row							
	Football athletes need to add a neck exercise.							

Table 11.4 Explosive Peak

Monday	Week 1		Week 2		Week 3		Week 4	
Hurdle warm-up	2 × 5		2 × 5		2 × 5		2 × 5	
Snatch squat	2 × 5		2 × 5		2 × 5		2 × 5	
1c. Power clean	4/3/2		4/3/2		4/3/2		4/3/2	
2c. Push jerk	4/3/2		4/3/2		4/3/2		4/3/2	
3. Hammer jammer extension	4/3/2		4/3/2		4/3/2		4/3/2	
**4. Pulling choice	3 × 10		3 × 10		3 × 10		3 × 10	
5. Biceps choice	3 × 10		3 × 10		3 × 10		3 × 10	
Thursday			**Unload**					
Hurdle warm-up	2 × 5		2 × 5		2 × 5		2 × 5	
Snatch squat	2 × 5		2 × 5		2 × 5		2 × 5	
1c. Power clean	4/3/2		4/3/2		4/3/2		4/3/2	
2c. Push jerk	4/3/2		4/3/2		4/3/2		4/3/2	
3. Hammer jammer extension	4/3/2		4/3/2		4/3/2		4/3/2	
**4. Pulling choice	3 × 10		3 × 10		3 × 10		3 × 10	
5. Biceps choice	3 × 10		3 × 10		3 × 10		3 × 10	
Date	**Comments**						**INT**	
	**4a. pull-ups, 4b. standing low row, 4c. lat pull-down, or 4d. bent-over row							
	Football athletes need to add a neck exercise.							

Rack Clean

To develop the explosive phase of the pull and learn how to get under the bar quickly

Start Position

With the bar resting on boxes or in a power rack, the athlete addresses the bar.

Procedure

1. Extend hips and knees explosively (figure 11.3a).
2. Simultaneously extend up on to the balls of the feet while shrugging the shoulders (figure 11.3b).
3. Pull yourself down and under the bar.
4. Jump feet out into a squatting stance (figure 11.3c).
5. Rotate elbows down and then up ahead of the bar.
6. Catch the bar on the front portion of the shoulders.
7. Flex the knees and hips to absorb the weight of the bar.

Key Points

- Don't pull with the arms before the body is completely extended.
- Extend up onto the balls of your feet and shrug the shoulders.

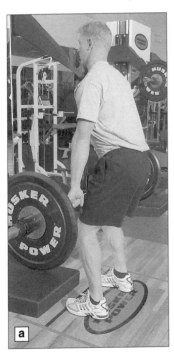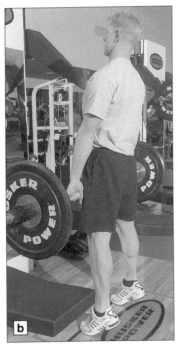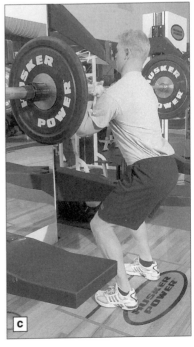

Figure 11.3 Rack clean.

Hang Clean

To develop the ability to express explosive power in the hips and legs

Start Position

1. See figure 11.4a.
2. Slowly extend the legs, elevating the bar to just above the knees.
3. As the bar passes the knees, extend the hips explosively.
4. The shoulders, hips, and knees should be in alignment with the bar held at arm's length and touching the top part of the thigh (figure 11.4b).

Procedure

1. Lower the bar to the top of the knees by flexing the hips (figure 11.4c).
2. Extend the hips explosively in a scooping action.
3. Simultaneously extend up on to the balls of the feet while shrugging the shoulders (figure 11.4d).
4. Pull yourself down and under the bar, leading with elbows pointed up.

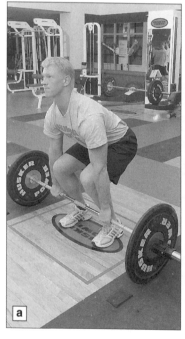
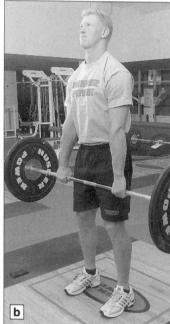
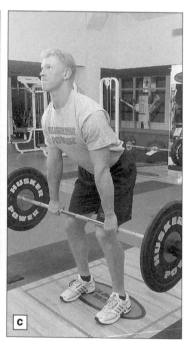

Figure 11.4 Hang clean.

5. Rotate elbows down and then up ahead of the bar.
6. Elevate the feet and move them out into a squatting stance.
7. Catch the bar on the front part of the shoulders.
8. Flex the knees and hips to absorb the weight of the bar (figure 11.4e).
9. Stand upright (figure 11.4f).

Key Points

- When the bar is lowered, don't hesitate at the top of the knees; extend the hips immediately. This lets you take advantage of the stretch-shortening cycle.
- The scooping action or a rebending of the legs can be compromised in two ways:
  1. By bending the arms at the elbows before the hips can be fully extended to the position shown in figure 11.4d.
  2. By swinging the bar away from the body.

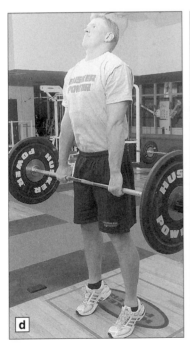
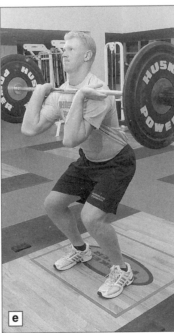
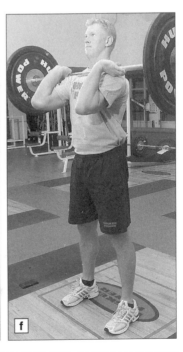

Power Clean

The clean uses a shoulder-width grip. The bar is pulled in one continuous motion and caught on the shoulders. The following are the five fundamental positions for the pulling action. It's difficult to observe and analyze this lift during normal execution. Videotape the execution of the lift and play it back in slow motion. Once the bar reaches a certain position, the video can be put on freeze frame so you analyze the fundamental positions.

Start Position
1. Place feet hip-width apart.
2. Bend legs with the lower leg touching the bar.
3. Place hands shoulder-width apart using an overhand grip.
4. Extend arms with elbows pointed out.
5. Fill chest with air and hold high.
6. Keep back flat.
7. Position shoulders just ahead of the bar.
8. Maintain head in a comfortable position.
9. See figure 11.5a.

First Pull
1. Extend the legs, elevating the bar to just above the knees.
2. During the movement of the bar from the floor to the knees, keep the angle of your back constant.
3. Don't jerk the bar off the floor—pull it smoothly and with control.
4. Keep the bar close to the legs.
5. Keep arms extended with elbows pointed out.
6. See figure 11.5b.

Second Pull
1. Extend hips up and forward explosively.
2. If you keep your arms straight, your knees will automatically flex or rebend as your hips extend. This movement is known as the double-knee bend or scooping action. This puts you in the position shown in figure 11.5c.
3. The bar should ride up the thighs.

Explosive Phase
1. Extend up onto the balls of the feet while simultaneously shrugging the shoulders.

2. During the explosive phase, the ankles, knees, and hips extend simultaneously, accelerating the bar upward. This is known as the triple extension. This puts you in the position in figure 11.5d.

3. Keep arms extended.

Receiving the Bar

1. Pull yourself down and under the bar.

2. Elevate the feet and move them out into a squatting stance.

3. Rotate elbows down and then up ahead of the bar.

4. Catch bar on the front portion of the shoulders.

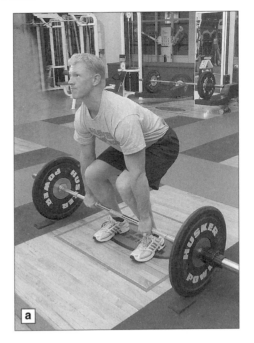

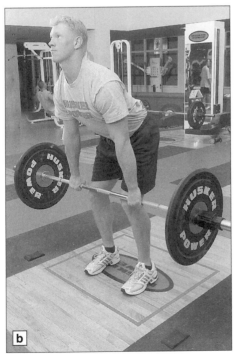

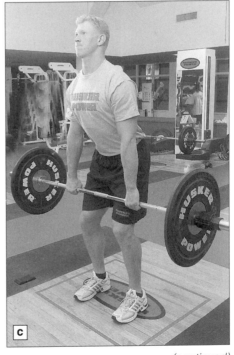

(continued)

Figure 11.5 Power clean.

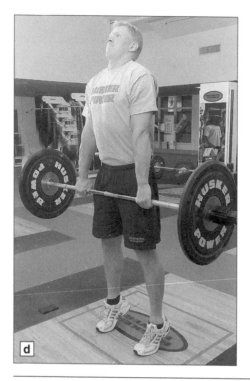 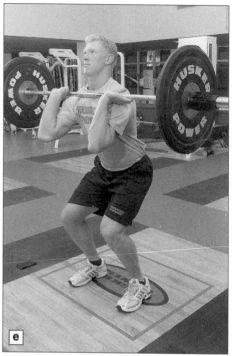

Figure 11.5 *(continued)*

5. Flex the knees and hips to absorb the weight of the bar.
6. Once the catch is made, stand to an erect position.
7. See figure 11.5e.

Key Points

- Don't pull with the arms before the body is completely extended. Be sure to extend up onto the balls of the feet and that the shoulders are kept shrugged; then pull yourself down and under the bar as quickly as possible.
- Elevate feet off the platform to help accelerate the body under the bar. As the feet are in the air, move them out into a squat stance to catch the bar. Be careful not to get the feet too wide.
- Steps 1 and 2 should occur simultaneously when receiving the bar.
- As the bar lands on the shoulders, throw the elbows up hard.
- Keep the chest up and back straight.

Standing Press

To strengthen the muscles of the shoulder girdle and teach the lifter to use the whole body while stabilizing weight overhead. This exercise can be used as an introductory lift for the power press.

Start Position

1. Place the bar in a rack at chest height.
2. Grip the bar a little wider than shoulder-width apart.
3. Place the bar behind the neck on the shoulders.
4. Stand in an erect position with feet shoulder-width apart (figure 11.6a).

Procedure

1. Press the bar overhead by extending the arms (figure 11.6b).
2. Lower the bar to start position.

Key Points

- Keep shoulders over the hips during the entire range of motion; don't let the shoulders drop back behind the hips.
- Place the feet as if you were going to perform a vertical jump, hip-width apart.
- When lowering the bar, simultaneously bend the knees as the bar hits the shoulders to help absorb the weight.

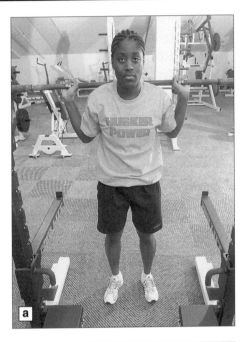

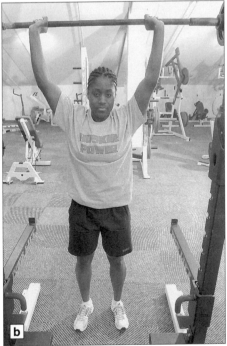

Figure 11.6 Standing press.

Power Press

To develop explosive power in the hips and legs and to strengthen the shoulder muscles. This exercise also develops the ability of the body to stabilize at the ankles, knees, hips, torso, shoulders, elbows, and wrists. If no jammer is available, use a bar.

Start Position
1. Place the bar behind the neck on the shoulders.
2. Stand in an erect position with feet shoulder-width apart.
3. Grip the bar a little wider than shoulder-width apart.

Procedure
1. Dip to a quarter-squat position.
2. Extend explosively onto the balls of the feet.
3. Press the bar by extending the arms completely.

Key Points
- Keep your torso perpendicular to the ground when lowering the bar; don't dip the torso forward.
- Complete the lift by pressing the bar with the legs straight. Don't drop under the bar on this exercise. Driving the legs will carry the bar to extension.

Push Jerk

To develop power in the hips and legs and to strengthen the shoulder muscles

Start Position
1. Place the bar behind the neck on the shoulders (figure 11.7a).
2. Stand in an erect position with feet hip-width apart.
3. Grip the bar with hands a little wider than shoulder-width apart.

Procedure
1. Dip straight down into a quarter-squat position (figure 11.7b).
2. Extend explosively onto the balls of the feet.
3. Drive the bar upward with the shoulders.
4. Push the body under the bar.
5. Split the legs apart as the feet leave the ground (figure 11.7c).

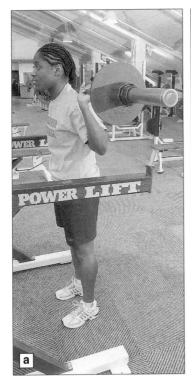 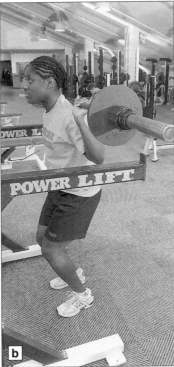 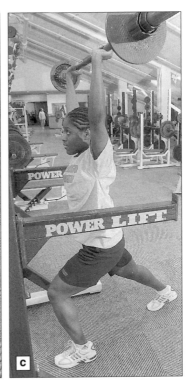

Figure 11.7 Push jerk.

6. Flex the front leg with the knee over the ankle.
7. Turn the front foot in slightly.
8. Bend the back leg slightly, with the back foot up on the toes.
9. Catch the bar overhead at arm's length by pressing upward.

Key Points

- Keep the body completely vertical during the entire movement. Any forward lean of the torso makes it difficult to complete the lift.
- The dip should be controlled, not rushed.
- Drive the bar up with the shoulders to take advantage of the power from the hips and legs. Gripping the bar lightly aids in driving the bar up with the shoulders instead of the arms. Push up on the bar only when the feet land on the ground. Pressing with the arms too soon won't let you take full advantage of the leg drive.
- The feet should be split straight forward and back; they should land on the ground hip-width apart.

Jammer Extension

To develop total body power by using a ground-based, multiple-joint movement. This exercise develops the ability of the body to stabilize at the ankles, knees, hips, torso, shoulders, elbows, and wrists.

Start Position

1. Grasp the handles with hands as close as possible (figure 11.8a).
2. Position shoulders directly behind hands as close as possible.
3. Place elbows at the side of the torso.
4. Position feet shoulder-width apart with heels off the ground.
5. Flex knees and hips.

Procedure

1. Rock back, then move forward to the start position to gain momentum.
2. Explode into the handles by extending at the hips, knees, and ankles onto the balls of the feet (figure 11.8b).
3. Follow through by extending the shoulders and elbows simultaneously.

Key Points

- Don't allow the shoulders to be positioned higher than the hands. If the shoulders are too high, the hips won't be flexed at the correct angle.
- When rocking back, keep the shoulders below the hands. This helps maintain the proper hip and knee flexion.

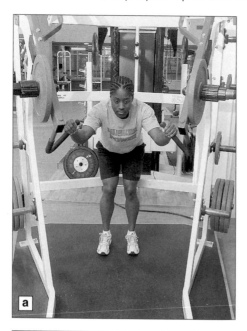 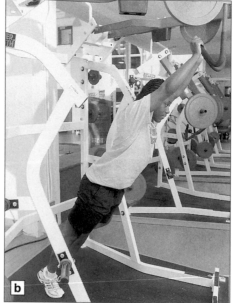

Figure 11.8 Jammer extension.

- Before you extend the hips, make sure the shoulders are close to the hands and the elbows are at the side of the torso.
- Position the body in a straight alignment from the feet to the hands at the finish of the exercise.

Pull-Ups

To strengthen the muscles of the upper back and abdominals and stretch the upper extremities

Start Position
Hang with a pronated grip and hands slightly wider than shoulders (figure 11.9a).

Procedure
1. Pull body up until the chin is even with the bar (figure 11.9b).
2. Return slowly to start position.

Key Points
- Keep legs stationary throughout the movement, avoiding any swinging motion.
- Return to the start position in a slow, controlled manner.
- Make sure to complete a full range of motion, experiencing a full stretch at the bottom of the exercise. Follow strength day repetitions.

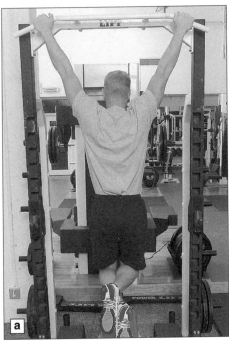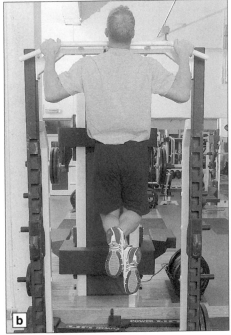

Figure 11.9 Pull-up.

Standing Low Row

To develop the muscles of the upper back

Start Position

1. Grasp handle with overhand grip (figure 11.10a).
2. Spread hands 6 to 12 inches apart.
3. Keep arms fully extended.
4. Stand with feet shoulder-width apart and knees slightly flexed.
5. Lean torso forward slightly.
6. Keep back flat.

Procedure

1. Pull the bar to the lower chest (figure 11.10b).
2. Slowly return the bar to arm's length and repeat.

Key Points

- Do this exercise slowly and smoothly. Don't lean forward or backward during the movement.
- When pulling the handle to the chest, squeeze the shoulder blades together. When returning the handle, feel the stretch in the back and shoulders. Visualize the muscles of the back stretching and squeezing during the movement. Follow strength day repetitions.

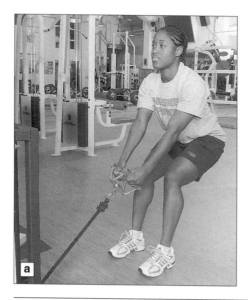 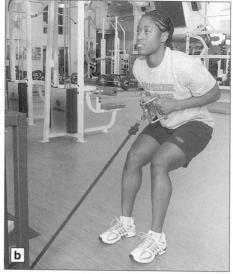

Figure 11.10   Standing low row.

Lat Pull-Down

To develop the muscles of the upper back

Start Position

1. Sit on a stool and anchor thighs under pads.
2. Using an overhand grip, place hands wider than shoulder-width apart (figure 11.11a).
3. Allow the weight to pull upward on the shoulders and upper back.

Procedure

1. Pull the bar down to the base of the neck (figure 11.11b).
2. Return the bar to start position with control; repeat.

Key Points

- When returning the bar to the start position, make sure to fully extend the arms so that you feel a stretch in the upper back.
- Keep back erect. Don't start the movement of the bar downward by leaning backward with the torso. This exercise should be done in a slow and controlled manner. Follow strength day repetitions.

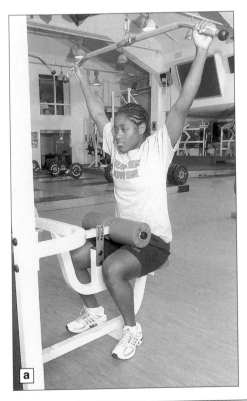 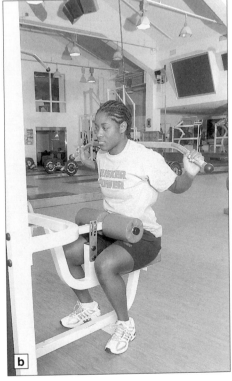

Figure 11.11 Lat pull-down.

Bent-Over Row

To develop the muscles of the upper back

Start Position

1. Stand with feet shoulder-width apart.
2. Grasp the bar with an overhand grip (figure 11.12a).
3. Spread hands 14 to 18 inches apart.
4. Bend forward at the waist until back is parallel to the floor.
5. Keep knees slightly bent.

Procedure

1. Pull the bar to the lower chest (figure 11.12b).
2. Lift elbows straight up and slightly outward.
3. Lower the bar under control; repeat.

Key Points

- Bar should be barely lifted off the floor before starting the exercise.
- When lowering the bar, keep back flat and feel a stretch in the upper back. When raising the bar, squeeze shoulder blades together. Follow strength day repetitions.

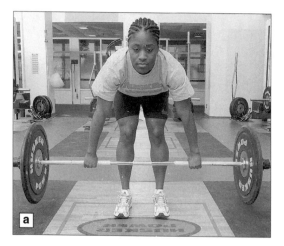 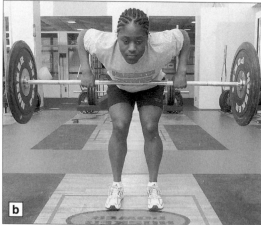

Figure 11.12 Bent-over row.

Biceps Choice

To develop the biceps

Start Position

1. Use an underhand grip with hands slightly wider than shoulder-width apart (figure 11.13a).
2. Position feet shoulder-width apart.
3. Hold at arm's length.

Procedure

1. Pull the bar or machine handle slowly to the shoulders by bending at the elbows (figure 11.13b).
2. Lower the bar in a controlled manner to the start position.
3. Keep the elbows positioned at the sides throughout the movement.

Key Point

- You can do this exercise with a barbell or a low-pulley machine. Follow strength day repetitions.

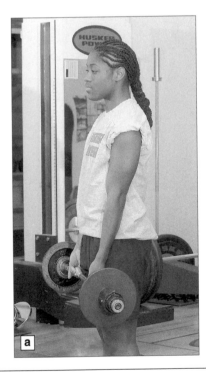 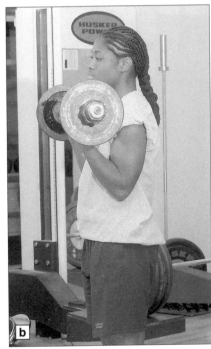

Figure 11.13 Biceps choice.

Strength Exercises

The recommended off-season strength day programs are shown in tables 11.5–11.8. These traditional lifts have provided great results for thousands of programs all over the country for many years. Remember that athletes tend to make better gains when they first begin lifting. Advanced athletes who have been lifting for several years sometimes struggle to make additional gains. The metabolic circuit is presented for advanced athletes in place of the traditional strength exercises. Athletes doing the metabolic circuit continue to do the explosive day exercises twice a week.

Squat

RDL (Romanian deadlift), clean deadlift, walking lunge

Bench press or incline press

Shoulder raises or shoulder press

Choice of triceps exercises

Push–pull circuit

Metabolic circuit (for advanced athletes)

Table 11.5 Recommended Strength Day Program

Exercise 1	*6. Squat (could alternate with front squat)	
Exercise 2	**Back and leg progression**	
	Base	7a. RDL
	Development	7b. Clean deadlift
	Peak	7c. ***Walking lunge with DBs
Exercise 3	***8a. Bench press or 8b. Incline press**	
Exercise 4	**Shoulder progression**	
	Base	9a. Shoulder raises
	Development	9b. Shoulder press
	Peak	9c. ***Shoulder press
Exercise 5	****10. Choice of triceps exercise**	
Exercise 6	11. Push–pull circuit	Two sets of 10 in off-season, 1 set of 10 in-season with lighter weights

*Test and determine strength levels on these major exercises.

**For triceps choice, use three sets of 10 throughout the program.

***In the peak phase for walking lunge and shoulder press, use three sets of 5 on each side.

Add choice of ab work at the end of the workout.

If no push–pull circuit, do jammer press for incline action, walking lunge with plate side-to-side for horizontal action, and bent-over row for decline action.

For advanced athletes, see metabolic strength day circuit.

Young athletes need to use a weight light enough to do at least 6 reps but not more than 15.

Table 11.6 Strength Base

Tuesday	Week 1		Week 2		Week 3		Week 4	
Hurdle warm-up	2 × 5		2 × 5		2 × 5		2 × 5	
Snatch squat	2 × 5		2 × 5		2 × 5		2 × 5	
6. Squat	3 × 10		3 × 10		3 × 10		3 × 10	
7a. RDL	3 × 10		3 × 10		3 × 10		3 × 10	
8a. Bench or 8b. Incline press	3 × 10		3 × 10		3 × 10		3 × 10	
9a. Shoulder raises	3 × 10		3 × 10		3 × 10		3 × 10	
10. Triceps exercise	3 × 10		3 × 10		3 × 10		3 × 10	
11. Push–pull circuit	2 × 10		2 × 10		2 × 10		2 × 10	
Friday				**Unload**				
Hurdle warm-up	2 × 5		2 × 5		2 × 5		2 × 5	
Snatch squat	2 × 5		2 × 5		2 × 5		2 × 5	
6. Squat	3 × 10		3 × 10		3 × 10		3 × 10	
7a. RDL	3 × 10		3 × 10		3 × 10		3 × 10	
8a. Bench or 8b. Incline press	3 × 10		3 × 10		3 × 10		3 × 10	
9a. Shoulder raises	3 × 10		3 × 10		3 × 10		3 × 10	
10. Triceps exercise	3 × 10		3 × 10		3 × 10		3 × 10	
11. Push–pull circuit	2 × 10		2 × 10		2 × 10		2 × 10	
Date			**Comments**					**INT**

Table 11.7 Strength Development

Tuesday	Week 1		Week 2		Week 3		Week 4	
Hurdle warm-up	2 × 5		2 × 5		2 × 5		2 × 5	
Snatch squat	2 × 5		2 × 5		2 × 5		2 × 5	
6. Squat	3 × 5		3 × 5		3 × 5		3 × 5	
7b. Clean deadlift	3 × 5		3 × 5		3 × 5		3 × 5	
8a. Bench or 8b. Incline press	3 × 5		3 × 5		3 × 5		3 × 5	
9b. Shoulder press	3 × 5		3 × 5		3 × 5		3 × 5	
10. Triceps exercise	3 × 10		3 × 10		3 × 10		3 × 10	
11. Push–pull circuit	2 × 10		2 × 10		2 × 10		2 × 10	
Friday				**Unload**				
Hurdle warm-up	2 × 5		2 × 5		2 × 5		2 × 5	
Snatch squat	2 × 5		2 × 5		2 × 5		2 × 5	
6. Squat	3 × 5		3 × 5		3 × 5		3 × 5	
7b. Clean deadlift	3 × 5		3 × 5		3 × 5		3 × 5	
8a. Bench or 8b. Incline press	3 × 5		3 × 5		3 × 5		3 × 5	
9b. Shoulder press	3 × 5		3 × 5		3 × 5		3 × 5	
10. Triceps exercise	3 × 10		3 × 10		3 × 10		3 × 10	
11. Push–pull circuit	2 × 10		2 × 10		2 × 10		2 × 10	
Date		**Comments**						**INT**

Table 11.8 Strength Peak

Tuesday	Week 1		Week 2		Week 3		Week 4	
Hurdle warm-up	2 × 5		2 × 5		2 × 5		2 × 5	
Snatch squat	2 × 5		2 × 5		2 × 5		2 × 5	
6. Squat	10\2		10\2		10\2		10\2	
7c. Walking lunge with DBs	3 × 5		3 × 5		3 × 5		3 × 5	
8a. Bench or 8b. Incline press	10\2		10\2		10\2		10\2	
9c. Shoulder press	3 × 5		3 × 5		3 × 5		3 × 5	
10. Triceps exercise	3 × 10		3 × 10		3 × 10		3 × 10	
11. Push–pull circuit	2 × 10		2 × 10		2 × 10		2 × 10	
Friday	**Unload**							
Hurdle warm-up	2 × 5		2 × 5		2 × 5		2 × 5	
Snatch squat	2 × 5		2 × 5		2 × 5		2 × 5	
6. Squat	10\2		10\2		10\2		10\2	
7c. Walking lunge with DBs	3 × 5		3 × 5		3 × 5		3 × 5	
8a. Bench or 8b. Incline press	10\2		10\2		10\2		10\2	
9c. Shoulder press	3 × 5		3 × 5		3 × 5		3 × 5	
10. Triceps exercise	3 × 10		3 × 10		3 × 10		3 × 10	
11. Push–pull circuit	2 × 10		2 × 10		2 × 10		2 × 10	
Date	**Comments**							**INT**

Squat

To develop the quadriceps, thigh adductors, gluteus maximus, and hamstrings. When done correctly, full squats strengthen the muscles, ligaments, and tendons that surround the knee. The core muscles are developed to a large degree in keeping the torso erect. The squat is the best exercise to develop lean body mass.

Start Position

1. Place the bar on the rack at chest height.
2. Position hands on the bar slightly wider than shoulder-width apart.
3. Step under the bar with feet parallel and knees slightly bent.
4. Position the bar comfortably on the shoulders in one of two positions:

   For a low bar squat, the bar sits across the scapula.

   For a high bar squat, the bar is one inch below the top of the shoulders across the traps (figure 11.14a).
5. Pull the shoulder blades together tightly.
6. Keep hips in vertical alignment with shoulders.
7. Lift the bar out of rack by extending the knees.
8. Step backward in as few steps as possible.
9. Position feet so they're parallel with toes pointed out slightly.
10. Keep heels slightly wider than the hips.

Procedure

1. Focus eyes directly ahead with head slightly up.
2. Take a deep breath and hold it.
3. Slowly lower the bar with control by bending at the hips and knees (figure 11.14b).
4. Keep the knees pointed out in alignment with the feet.
5. The instant the thighs are parallel to the ground, explode out of the bottom position.
6. Keep the back flat and shoulder blades drawn together.
7. Keep your weight back on your heels.
8. Don't throw the head back.
9. Exhale your breath as you near the completion of the lift.
10. Complete the squat by fully extending the knees and hips.

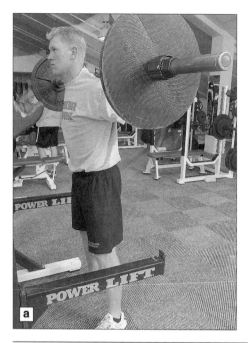 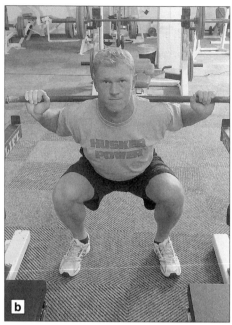

Figure 11.14 Squat.

Key Points

- Make sure the bar is in a good solid position on the shoulders by pulling the shoulder blades together tightly.
- The closer you position your hands together on the bar, the tighter you can pull the shoulder blades together.
- Use a stance that's most comfortable to allow proper depth.
- Control is the most important factor—don't try to bounce out of the bottom.
- If you try to recover to an upright position after bouncing out of the bottom, your hips will rise too quickly and cause your back to round out. This takes the stress off the legs and puts it on the lower back. Take extra care to descend slowly and with control.
- Keep shoulder blades together. If the shoulder blades relax, the lower back rounds out.
- Pick out a spot on the wall in front of you. Keep eyes focused on that spot throughout the performance of the squat. This helps keep the body in a stable position and control the bar. If eyes are looking all over the place, you have a better chance of losing balance. Squat inside the rack or use two or three spotters.
- Flex the knees and hips.

RDL

To develop the upper hamstrings, gluteus maximus, and erector stabilizers. You can do this exercise as an introductory lift for hang cleans.

Start Position

1. Grip the bar a little wider than shoulder-width apart.
2. Stand in an erect position with feet hip-width apart as if you're going to perform a vertical jump (figure 11.15a).
3. Keep toes pointed straight or slightly angled out.

Procedure

1. Fill chest with air and hold high.
2. Unlock knees and bend forward.
3. Move hips backward as the bar is lowered (figure 11.15b).
4. Lower the bar until hips can't go back any farther.
5. Raise the bar by extending hips forward to start position.
6. Keep back flat with a slight arch in lower back.

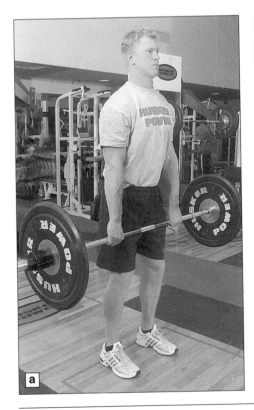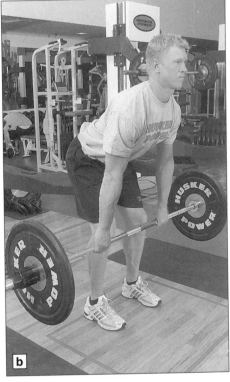

Figure 11.15 RDL.

Clean Deadlift

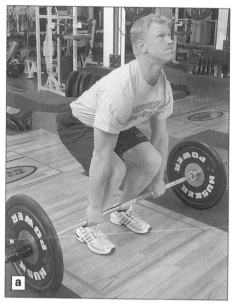

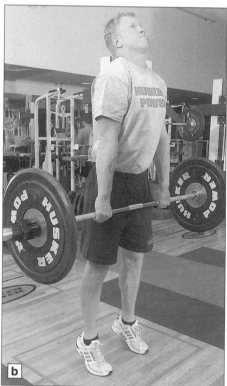

To learn how to lift the bar off the ground properly and to develop the leg, hip, back, and trapezius muscles.

Start Position

With the bar resting on the floor or a platform, address the bar with a clean grip (figure 11.16a).

Procedure

1. Slowly extend the legs, elevating the bar to just above the knees.
2. Extend the hips forward and up.
3. The shoulders, hips, and knees should be in alignment as the lift is completed (figure 11.16b).
4. During the movement of the bar from the floor to the knees, keep the angle of the back constant. The shoulders, hips, and bar move together as a unit.
5. Don't jerk the bar off the floor; pull it smoothly and with control.
6. Keep the bar close to the legs. From above the knees, the bar should ride up the thighs.
7. Keep the back flat with lower back slightly arched.

Figure 11.16 Clean deadlift.

Walking Lunge

To strengthen the muscles of the hips, legs, and trunk

Start Position

1. Start in a standing position with dumbbells at sides.
2. Keep arms straight down, palms in.

Procedure

1. Take an exaggerated step forward with one leg (figure 11.17a).
2. Drop hips straight down until the front thigh is parallel to the floor (figure 11.17b).
3. Maintain balance as you push off and step through with the back leg.
4. Repeat the step forward with the opposite leg until you complete the set.

Key Points

- Make sure that hips and shoulders remain square throughout the exercise.
- Don't bounce in the bottom position.
- This exercise can be modified to put more emphasis on the hips by taking a smaller step and leaning forward so that the arms hang, with the weight in line with the front foot. The weights should touch the floor to allow full range of motion and stability.

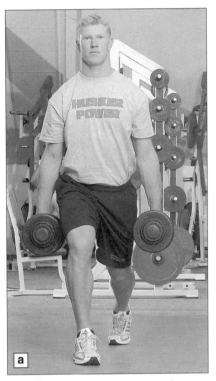

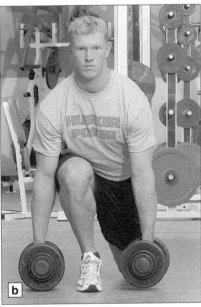

Figure 11.17 Walking lunge.

Bench Press

To develop the pectoral muscles, with some development of the anterior deltoids and triceps

Start Position

1. Place feet flat on the ground.
2. Slightly arch back as buttocks are set on the bench.
3. Pull the shoulder blades inward as you push the chest upward.
4. Grip the bar with hands slightly wider than shoulder-width apart.
5. Position yourself so the bar is lined up with the top of your head.
6. Take the bar from the rack with the aid of a spotter.
7. Position the bar over chest (figure 11.18a).

Procedure

1. Take a deep breath and hold your chest high.
2. Lower the bar slowly and under control.
3. Allow the bar to just touch the chest at about nipple level (figure 11.18b).
4. Drive the bar explosively off the chest.
5. The movement of the bar should be up and slightly back.
6. Exhale as you lock the bar out to full arm's length.

Key Points

- Grip the bar so that when it touches the chest the elbow joint is at about a 90-degree angle.

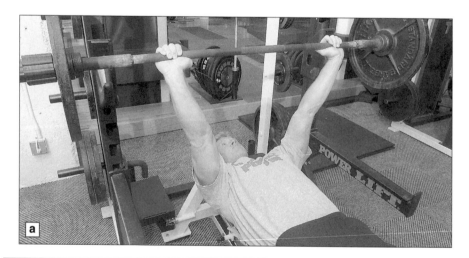

Figure 11.18 Bench press.

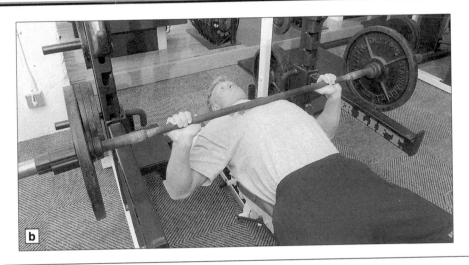

Figure 11.18 *(continued)*

- The spotter and the lifter work together in a coordinated effort to guide the bar into a lifting position and get it racked. The spotter should also have his or her hands under the bar and be constantly alert.
- It's a good idea for beginners to have the thumbs wrapped around the bar.
- Many times the lift is not completed because the athlete gets the bar out of the groove. The most common error is to let the bar come off the chest moving toward the legs. This movement takes the bar out of the groove. The bar must come straight up and back off the chest so that maximum force can be applied to the bar.

Incline Press

To develop the upper pectoral muscles, the anterior deltoids, and triceps

Start Position

1. Place feet flat on the ground.
2. Slightly arch back as buttocks are set on the bench.
3. Pull the shoulder blades inward as you push the chest upward.
4. Grip bar with hands slightly wider than shoulder-width apart.
5. Make sure thumbs are wrapped around the bar.
6. Position yourself so that the bar is lined up with the top of your head.
7. Take the bar from the rack with the aid of a spotter (figure 11.19a).
8. Position the bar over chest.

Procedure

1. Take a deep breath and hold chest high.

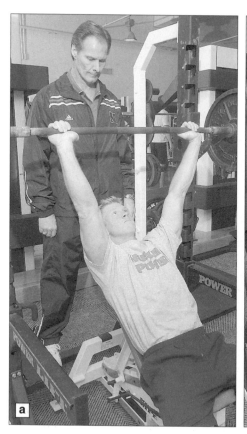
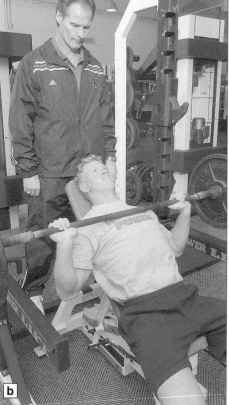

Figure 11.19 Incline press.

2. Lower the bar slowly and with control.
3. Allow the bar to just touch the upper chest at the base of the neck (figure 11.19b).
4. Drive the bar explosively off the chest.
5. Move the bar up and slightly back.
6. Exhale as you lock the bar out to full arm's length.

Key Points

- Grip the bar so that when it touches the chest the elbow joint is at about a 90-degree angle.
- The spotter and the lifter work together in a coordinated effort to guide the bar into a lifting position and get it racked. The spotter should also have his or her hands under the bar and be constantly alert.
- Wrap your thumbs around the bar.

Front Shoulder Raises

To isolate and develop the anterior or front deltoid muscles

Start Position

1. Stand with dumbbells in each hand held at the front of thighs.
2. Use an overhand grip.
3. Extend arms.
4. Keep feet about hip-width apart.

Procedure

1. Raise both dumbbells upward and forward until they're at shoulder level (figure 11.20).
2. Lower dumbbells and repeat.

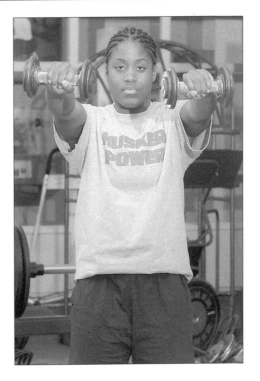

Figure 11.20 Front shoulder raises.

Lateral Shoulder Raises

To isolate and develop the lateral deltoid muscles

Start Position

1. Stand with dumbbells in each hand held at the side of the thighs.
2. Use an overhand grip.
3. Extend arms.
4. Keep feet about hip-width apart.

Procedure

1. Raise both dumbbells upward and sideways until they're at shoulder level (figure 11.21).
2. Lower dumbbells and repeat.

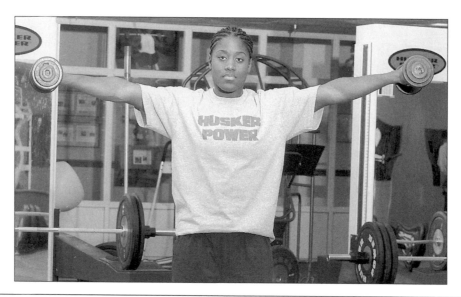

Figure 11.21 Lateral shoulder raises.

Bent-Over Shoulder Raises

To isolate and develop the posterior or back deltoid muscles

Start Position

1. Use an overhand grip.
2. Keep feet about hip-width apart.
3. Bend at the hips until the back is parallel to the ground.
4. Extend arms, hanging them straight down.

Procedure

1. Raise both dumbbells upward and back until they're at shoulder level (figure 11.22).
2. Lower dumbbells and repeat.

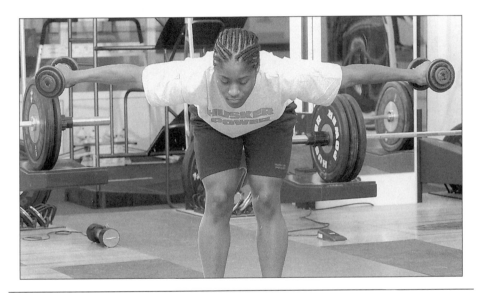

Figure 11.22   Bent-over shoulder raises.

Shoulder Press

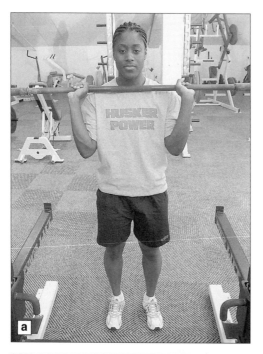

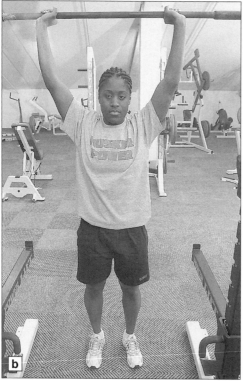

To strengthen the muscles of the shoulder girdle and teach lifters to use the whole body in the stabilizing of weight overhead. You can use this exercise as an introductory lift for the power press.

Start Position

1. Place the bar in a rack at chest height.
2. Grip the bar with hands a little wider than shoulder-width apart.
3. Place the bar on the upper chest (figure 11.23a).
4. Stand in an erect position with feet shoulder-width apart.

Procedure

1. Press the bar overhead by extending the arms (figure 11.23b).
2. Lower the bar to start position.

Key Points

- Keep shoulders over hips during the entire range of motion.
- Stand with feet hip-width apart, positioned as if you were about to do a vertical jump.
- When lowering the bar, simultaneously bend the knees as the bar hits the shoulders to help absorb the weight.

Figure 11.23 Shoulder press.

Triceps Pushdown

To develop the triceps

Start Position

1. Stand with feet flat on floor.
2. Position hands on pull-down bar about six inches apart.
3. Use an overhand grip.
4. Pull the bar down to extended arm position.

Procedure

1. Allow the bar to rise until there's a 90-degree angle at the elbows (figure 11.24a).
2. Push the bar down until arms are extended (figure 11.24b).
3. Keep elbows at the sides throughout the movement.

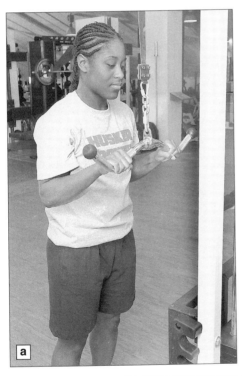
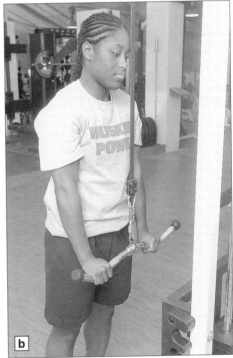

Figure 11.24   Triceps pushdown.

Push–Pull Circuit

The objective of core training is to improve performance and reduce soft tissue injuries of the lower back, hips, and legs. There's some confusion about which muscle groups actually constitute the core. Most coaches consider the abdominal muscle group as the core muscles and have athletes do hundreds of sit-ups, leg lifts, and similar exercises with the pelvis on the ground.

The core muscles actually consist of all the muscles that control the pelvis and trunk joints attached to the pelvic girdle. The core includes 35 muscles on each side of the body and provides core stabilization and equilibrium for the entire body.

The pelvis is the seat of power that connects the upper body to the lower body. The origins of the largest, most powerful muscles are attached to the pelvis, which provides leverage for total body movements in all planes of motion. The pelvis acts in union with the sacrum as a foundation for the trunk, allowing for the upright posture of the human body. The pelvis also functions as a relay station to transmit the ground reaction forces from the legs to the upper body. Thus, the pelvis is not only the seat of power but also the control center for maintaining the body's equilibrium.

The Hammer Strength push–pull circuit trains the core in a functional way with the body standing in an upright position. Unlike sit-ups or core exercises with the pelvis stabilized by the ground, the push–pull exercises require the core muscles to provide stabilization of the pelvis in the standing position. While standing, the athlete's pelvis and trunk must be stabilized by core muscles to provide equilibrium for the body to perform the exercise. Everyone realizes that athletic functional movements aren't done from a seated position. If seated during exercise, the athlete's pelvis and trunk don't have to be stabilized to perform the exercise, and as a result little carryover for athletic performance is achieved.

- *Ground base.* For movement to occur, the body relies not only on its own muscle power but on external forces, such as gravity. If our bodies were floating in space, we wouldn't be able to move even a whisker, regardless of the amount of muscular force we tried to express. The arms and legs would just flail. To express maximum force, you must have your feet on the ground. Muscular force is exerted against the ground, with the feet causing an equal and opposite reaction in the direction of the movement. With the push–pull exercises, the feet are anchored to the ground to provide stability while the hip and shoulder joints provide mobility.

- *Reciprocal actions.* Reciprocal action means one side of the body extends as the opposite side flexes. The Hammer Strength push–pull machines use reciprocal actions. As one side of the body pushes or extends, the opposite side pulls or flexes, strengthening the body in a functional way. When you run, you don't use just one side of your body. Reciprocal action, such as walking and running, are initiated by the leg and hip muscles extending and causing an equal and opposite ground force reaction. As the hips, knees, and ankles extend, the ground reaction force is transmitted to the trunk muscles so that the opposite leg can swing forward. We developed the push–pull circuit by accident. We cut the seat off a Hammer Strength seated row trying to get a machine that our wrestlers could use standing up. When the row failed to work as we wanted, I called Gary Jones and explained what we'd done to his machine. He came right over. He literally jumped into his airplane and flew to Lincoln. After looking at the machine cut into pieces, he took the pieces to our tool room and welded a Z-shaped base piece that had originally been a straight piece. He then turned the lever arm around backward. With the new arrangement, the lever arms were offset or staggered. As a result, we had the first reciprocal machine with a left-arm push and a right-arm pull. He then made a machine to match with the lever arms reversed so the right arm pushed and the left arm pulled. We called them the "Twist Right" and the "Twist Left," and our wrestlers loved them. We had them for two years while the other four machines were developed, making up the six-station push–pull circuit.

- *Inner and outer core.* The core muscles consist of one inner unit group and three outer unit systems that couple the lower body with the upper body. Stability starts with the deep inner unit muscles, which are the primary stabilizers. The outer motor units help stabilize the pelvis, hips, and back and also power reciprocal actions.

For movement to occur, there must be stability, giving the joint a firm base from which to work. As Christopher Norris (2000) has written, "Stability of a joint implies the body's ability to control the entire range of motion around that joint." Weightlifters usually wear a belt to support their lower back and abdominal region. Wearing a belt stabilizes the trunk instead of the deep inner core muscles. The body becomes dependent on the belt instead of relying on the body's natural belt, the inner core muscles.

The inner unit consists of the transverse abdominis, multifidus, diaphragm, and pelvic floor. This unit forms a natural support system for the lower abdominal and back region (figure 11.25).

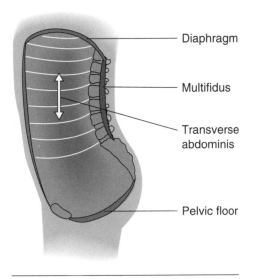

Figure 11.25 Pelvic girdle muscles of the inner unit.

If these muscles don't contract first, it's like having a car with wheels out of alignment. With the wheels out of alignment, some of the energy normally used to move the car is displaced, causing the whole car to vibrate. The body works the same way. If the inner unit is not stabilized, some of the energy is displaced, which causes the hip and trunk joints to twist awkwardly. Limb power is lost, and the joints are stressed, causing injury.

A process called abdominal hollowing or centering can help fire up the inner core muscles to achieve correct pelvic, hip, and trunk stability. Pull the belly button in and up toward the spine without taking a big breath. This causes the deep inner abdominal muscles to contract and stabilize the pelvis and spine. A way to feel this contraction is to imagine receiving a punch to the abdominal area. Forcibly blow some air out, as if you were coughing, as you pull your navel up and in. You should be able to hold this contracted position and breathe as you exercise. The strength of the deep inner muscles is not as important as their ability to contract first, prior to the outer unit muscles of the trunk.

The three outer unit systems are as follows:

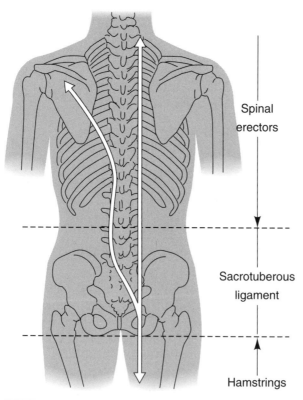

Figure 11.26   Pelvic girdle deep longitudinal system of the outer unit.

1. The deep longitudinal system, which consists of the hamstrings coupled with the spinal erectors via the sacrotuberous ligament. This system helps keep the body erect (figure 11.26).

2. The posterior oblique system, which consists of the gluteus maximus coupled with the latissimus dorsi on the opposite side of the body via the thoracodorsal fascia. This system aids in rotation of the spine and pelvis (figure 11.27).

3. The anterior oblique system, which consists of the thigh adductors, which couple with the external and internal

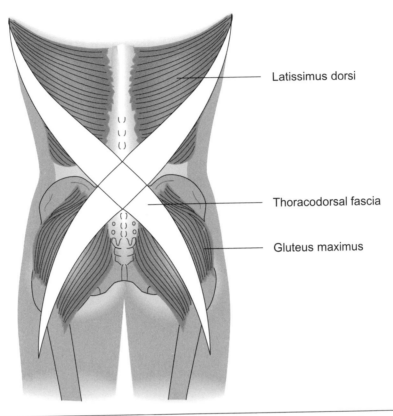

Latissimus dorsi

Thoracodorsal fascia

Gluteus maximus

Figure 11.27 Pelvic girdle posterior oblique system of the outer unit.

oblique via the abdominal fascia. This system aids in rotation of the spine and pelvis (figure 11.28).

Push–pull technique. Proper technique is necessary to derive the maximum benefits of performance enhancement and prevent possible injury. Keep in mind: technique before strength. Always make sure lifting form is correct before increasing the weight.

Control. Don't focus on the push or pull action by using the arms. Control the movement in both directions by keeping tension with the inner unit muscles doing the work and the power radiating outward to the arms.

Breathing. Inhale just before executing a lift, and hold it during the first phase of the exercise movement. As you return weight to the start position, breathe out forcibly. This keeps the deep inner abdominal muscles contracted during the exercise movement.

Full range of motion. If you want to receive the full benefits of strength training, you must execute all exercises through their full range of motion. Partial movements are unwise because over time the range of motion for the muscle is reduced. This can make the body part less flexible and

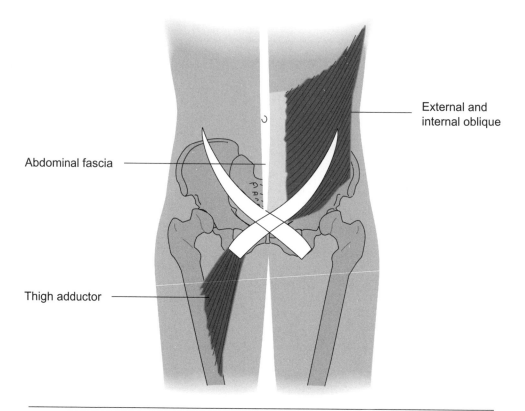

Figure 11.28 Pelvic girdle anterior oblique system of the outer unit.

increase the chances of pulling or straining a muscle. Perform exercises exactly as described.

Levels of difficulty. *Beginner level*—1 set of 10 reps done twice a week. Move from one station to the next to complete the circuit. It will take only a few minutes to complete all six stations. Rest as long as needed between stations. Performing one set following the traditional lifts during the in-season works great.

Intermediate level—After going through all six stations, rest as needed, then repeat all six stations. Do this twice a week.

Advanced level—Do three trips through all six stations with as much rest between stations and between sets as needed. Athletes should be fully recovered and ready for the next trip through the circuit within two or three minutes or less.

This type of training wires muscles to perform correctly. The push–pull circuit is considered part of a slow strength program and is not intended to replace explosive lifting for athletes. Athletes need to make a choice of square stance, neutral stance, or single-leg stance when performing the push–pull circuit. Nebraska recommends the square stance for athletes who have normal hip rotation and the single-leg stance for athletes who have problems with limited hip rotation.

Square Stance

The push–pull machines require a good base of support in a balanced position. This is accomplished by firmly positioning the feet flat on the ground. Position the feet directly beneath the hip joints perpendicular to the front base of the push–pull machine. Keep heels and toes in alignment and pointed straight ahead. Bend knees slightly and keep in alignment with feet. Bend hips slightly and keep squared directly above the feet. Keep shoulders squared with the feet and hips. Maintain even distribution of body weight on both feet. See figure 11.29.

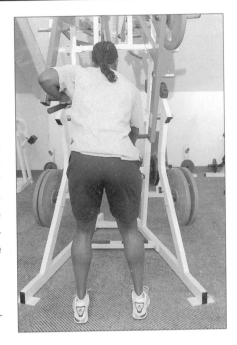

Figure 11.29 Square stance.

Neutral Stance

If you're pushing with the left side, position the left foot back with the toes of the left foot even with the heel of the right foot (figure 11.30). An imaginary line drawn from the front base of the push–pull machine passes to the back of the heel of the right foot and to the front of the toes of the left foot. Keep heels and toes in alignment and pointed straight ahead. Bend knees slightly and align with feet, which are pointed straight ahead. Bend hips slightly and keep parallel with feet. Position shoulders parallel to the feet and hips. Keep body weight evenly distributed on both feet.

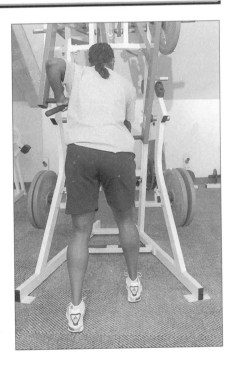

Figure 11.30 Neutral stance.

Procedure

1. Position feet in a square or neutral stance
2. Grasp handles of push–pull machine.
3. Bend knees and hips slightly, keeping weight distributed evenly on both feet.
4. Contract inner unit muscles by drawing belly button toward spine.
5. Push and pull keeping weight distributed evenly on both feet, as possible.
6. Initiate movement from the inner core and let force radiate out up to the arms.
7. Keep hips as steady as possible as the shoulders rotate. Imagine the shoulders and spine as a T, with the bottom of the T rotating on the pelvis.
8. Keep head centered between the feet.

Single-Leg Stance

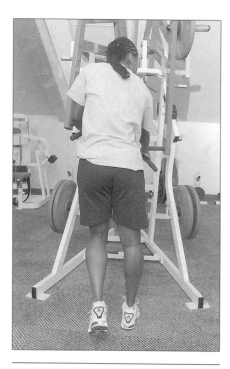

Figure 11.31 Single-leg stance.

When we're walking or running, the weight of our body transfers and shifts from one leg to the other. As the swing leg moves forward, the pelvis must rotate on the ground-based leg. The power to do this action comes from the extension of the ground-based leg via the outer unit muscles. The abdominal oblique and lower back muscles rotate the pelvis, moving the center of gravity forward. Place the left foot down to push–pull left and the right foot down to the push–pull right. Keep shoulders, hips, and knees parallel to the ground. Rotate the pelvis on the stationary femur head by rotating the swing foot around the stationary foot.

Procedure

1. Take a single-leg stance (figure 11.31). If using push–pull left, stand on the right leg. If using push–pull right, stand on the left leg.

2. Grasp the handles of the push–pull machine.

3. Bend knee and hip slightly, with foot centered between push–pull machine.

4. Contract inner unit muscles by drawing navel toward spine.

5. Push and pull, keeping weight centered over foot as much as possible.

6. Initiate movement from the inner core and let force radiate up to the arms. It's not necessary to use a heavy weight on this exercise. The movement is more important.

7. Rotate the pelvis on the femur head, keeping shoulders, hips, and knees parallel to the ground (see figure 11.32).

8. Keep swinging your foot an inch off the ground during the entire movement.

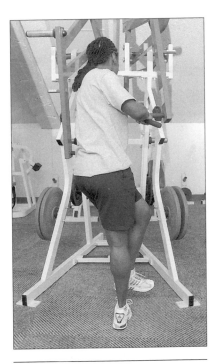

Figure 11.32 Pelvis rotation.

Metabolic Circuit for Advanced Athletes

We've seen this program make better increases in muscle mass and strength than traditional lifting programs. The problem is that it's extremely demanding. It's not for beginners, and even advanced athletes won't want to maintain this intensity for more than four to six weeks. The program increase metabolism, which burns more calories at rest. As the athletes build muscle, they lose fat. Use the metabolic circuit only during the base phase in the postseason or off-season. The metabolic circuit replaces the strength day on Tuesday and Friday, but the explosive day exercises continue to be on Monday and Thursday. The exercise order for the metabolic circuit is not critical except for the first station. The squat needs to be done first in this circuit or the program won't produce the desired results. The other eight exercises can be done in any order. Try to have one exercise for each large muscle in the body. The program should start with multiple-joint exercises and finish with single-joint exercises. Exercises using larger muscle groups release more testosterone. Some coaches alternate leg, chest, and back exercises to allow for recovery of muscle groups.

Husker Power Metabolic Circuit Stations

1. Squat—works thighs, hamstrings, hips, lower back
2. Lying leg curl—works hamstrings
3. Leg extension—works quads
4. Bench press—works chest, shoulders, triceps
5. Lat pull-down—works lats, biceps, forearms
6. Shoulder press—works shoulders, triceps
7. Low lat pull-down—works lats, biceps, forearms
8. Triceps extension—works triceps
9. Biceps curl—works biceps

Load and time. Use a weight that allows for a set of 10 repetitions. Allow 80 seconds total for the work and rest at each station. Each rep takes about 2 seconds. The squat takes longer, but for most of the exercises most of the 80 seconds is used for recovery. More growth hormone is released when the number of repetitions is 10 as opposed to 5 or fewer, and more is released when the rest period is at 1 minute rather than 3 or 4 minutes. The speed of each movement is not explosive but is done under control to allow good form. Note that all sets are done at each station before rotating to the next station. This is different from the push–pull circuit in which athletes move from station to station and then repeat the circuit.

Levels of difficulty. *Beginner*—1 set of 10 reps done 2 or 3 days per week. Be sure to have a physician's clearance, and present the release form to the supervisor before attempting this program. Allow 80 seconds to complete each station.

Intermediate—The program should be progressive in nature and advance to two sets at each station before moving to the next station. The circuit is done twice a week on strength day.

Advanced—Three sets at each station with higher loads to increase strength and bone density. Multiple sets work best for development of strength and local muscular endurance. The gains made will be at a faster rate than gains achieved through single- or double-set programs. Total time is 36 minutes.

The metabolic circuit should not be used year round. The advanced level (three sets) is very advanced and should only be used during the base phase to develop lean muscle. The advanced level should not be done by young athletes, who don't have enough strength.

The following chart shows the 14 pounds of muscle developed by Kyle Vanden Bosch as he prepared for his senior year in college. Kyle is a professional football player now, and this chart shows his progress doing the advanced level Husker Power metabolic circuit. Kyle was voted the Lifter of the Year as a junior and was looking for a program that would bring additional results. Nationally recognized scientist Dr. Bill Kraemer visited Nebraska many years ago when he was a strength coach at Carroll College in Iowa. I put him through a circuit workout that was so hard it about killed him. We called it the "Death Circuit" then but changed the name to the "Survivor Circuit" to give it a more positive spin, but it was still so hard that we quit using it. However, 15 years after first trying the workout, Dr. Kraemer kept tweaking it. When he felt he had something to share, he called and explained how the program built up too much lactic acid in the muscle and was too painful for athletes to handle. The metabolic circuit corrects that and also sends a growth hormone throughout the body to produce strength and size gains.

We needed someone tough to handle the circuit, so we asked our strongest athlete, Kevin Coleman, to give it a try. He had just won the national championship in the shot-put as a junior and was looking for a program to take him to another level. Within a very few weeks, Kevin made gains he hadn't imagined possible, so we asked him to address the football team. He told the Nebraska players they weren't tough enough to handle this program. We challenged 30 players to sign up to do the metabolic circuit, but we warned them it was all or nothing. Once they committed to the six-week program, they could not back out. We also required them to be upper classmen. The program increases strength rapidly, but we've learned over time not to put some athletes on the circuit because it makes them gain weight so quickly. For example, Lawrence Phillips was a powerful 205-pound I-Back who did the program for four weeks before we pulled him off it at 226 pounds.

Vanden Bosch Progress Chart

Weight	Muscle	10-yard dash	40-yard dash	Agility run	Vertical jump (in.)
262	229	1.67 (E)	4.85 (E)	4.09 (E)	32
267	243	1.7 (E)	4.84 (E)	3.97 (E)	32.5
5	**14**	**0.03**	**-0.01**	**-0.12**	**0.5**

Landing Drills for Women

Coaches often wonder whether female athletes should lift the same way as male athletes. The only difference in lifting programs for female athletes are the landing drills that are recommended to strengthen the knee. Orthopedic doctors recommend these exercises be included for women. The purpose of the landing drills is to develop proper jumping and landing techniques. There are four phases of the landing drills that require special attention: the start position, the countermovement, the jump, and the actual landing.

Be sure to use an area that's firm yet has some resiliency, such as a hard rubber mat. You'll need a box for some of the drills. Choose two or three drills for each explosive lifting day. Drills are in order of difficulty. Start with easier drills and progress to the tougher ones. Select shoes with great support. Female athletes may want to try the shoes designed specifically for them by adidas. The A3 Anthene provides great overall support, and the Assured has a midfoot strap for medial and lateral support.

Phase 1: Correct Posture and Body Alignment Before Jumping

- Keep head vertical, chin up, eyes focused forward.
- Keep back straight by drawing shoulder blades together.
- Keep lower back slightly arched.
- Keep the knees unlocked.
- Stand with feet parallel about hip-width apart with toes pointed straight ahead.

Avoid

- Spacing feet too wide
- Rounding the lower back with shoulders rolled forward

Phase 2: The Countermovement

- Perform this phase quickly.
- Squat by bending at the hips, knees, and ankles four to six inches.
- Drop shoulders forward slightly during the squatting phase so that knees and shoulders are directly above toes.
- Swing arms back behind hips during the squat phase.

Avoid

- Leaning forward too much
- Bending the hips, knees, and ankles too much
- Moving too slowly

Phase 3: The Jump

- Reverse direction of the countermovement quickly.
- Drive off toes actively against the ground.
- Thrust arms upward directly overhead.

Avoid

- Pausing at the bottom of the countermovement

Key Terms

Explode

Drive off toes

Straight as an arrow

Phase 4: Soft Landings

- Land with feet nearly flat (balls of feet touch first, then heel).
- Bend at the knees and hips (try to stop the flexion of knees as quickly as possible).
- Keep shoulders and knees directly over toes.
- Be able to land and hold position for two to five seconds without losing balance.

Avoid

- Landing on heels
- Knees adduct inward
- Bending at knees and hips more than necessary
- Losing balance

Key Terms

Shock absorber

Light as a feather

Drop Jump

To learn how to land and to strengthen the legs and hips

Procedure

1. Stand with feet parallel about hip-width apart (figure 11.33a).
2. Step off the box, landing on balls of feet.
3. Flex knees and hips; hold for a five-second count (figure 11.33b).
4. Relax legs and immediately get on box for next repetition.
5. Do five repetitions.

Key Point

- Start with a box that's 24 inches high and gradually work up to greater heights as strength increases. It's not necessary to use boxes higher than 42 inches.

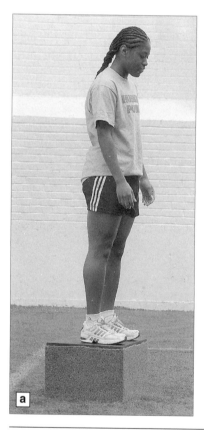 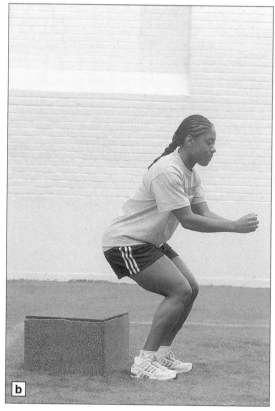

Figure 11.33 Drop jump.

Vertical Jump

To develop explosive power

Procedure

1. Stand with feet parallel about hip-width apart.
2. Use a countermovement by dipping four to six inches and then jump.
3. Swing both arms straight up and reach as high as you can (figure 11.34).
4. Do five jumps and record the best jump (total height).

Key Point

- Don't take any steps before jumping.

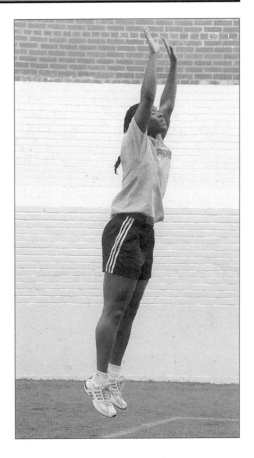

Figure 11.34 Vertical jump.

Tuck Jump

To learn how to land, to develop explosive power, and to prepare the body for more intense power drills

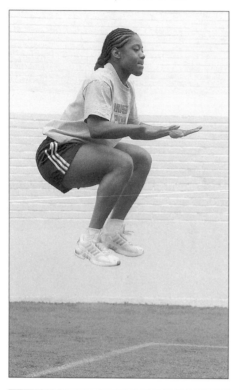

Figure 11.35 Tuck jump.

Procedure

1. Stand with feet parallel about hip-width apart.
2. Use a countermovement by dipping four to six inches and then jump.
3. Bring knees up to the chest as high you can (figure 11.35).
4. Land as softly as possible and hold the landing position for five seconds before the next repetition.
5. Do five repetitions.

Key Points

- Don't take any steps before jumping.
- Hold hands palms down at chest height and attempt to touch with knees.
- Visualize landing like a shock absorber.

180-Degree Jump

To learn how to land, to develop explosive power, and to prepare the body for more intense power drills

Procedure

1. Stand with feet parallel about hip-width apart.
2. Use a countermovement by dipping four to six inches (figure 11.36a).
3. Explosively jump up by simultaneously swinging the arms forward and extending the legs (figure 11.36b).
4. While in the air, rotate 180 degrees.
5. After contact, hold landing for two seconds (figure 11.36c) and then rotate 180 degrees in the opposite direction.
6. Do five repetitions.

Key Points

1. Jump with both feet.
2. Rotate in the air.
3. Land softly on two feet and hold for two seconds.

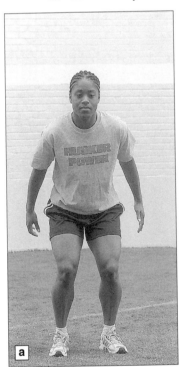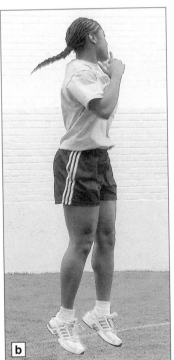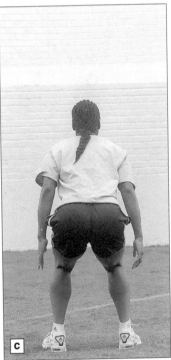

Figure 11.36 180-degree jump.

Broad Jump and Vertical Jump

To learn how to land, to develop explosive power, and to prepare the body for more intense power drills

Procedure

1. Stand with feet parallel about hip-width apart.
2. Swing arms backward and bend at knees and hips (figure 11.37a).
3. Explosively jump up and forward (45 degree angle) by simultaneously swinging the arms forward and extending the legs (figure 11.37b).
4. While in the air, pull knees up toward the body.
5. Jump for as much distance as possible.
6. Land as softly as possible and hold the landing position for five seconds (figure 11.37c).
7. Repeat three broad jumps (up and forward) and then do a vertical jump (figure 11.37d).
8. Do five repetitions.

Key Points

- Jump with both feet.
- Hold each jump for a count of five.

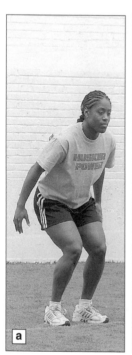 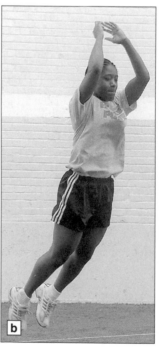 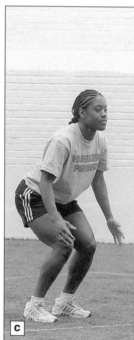 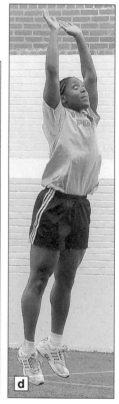

Figure 11.37 Broad jump and vertical jump.

Depth Jumps

To develop explosive vertical movements

Procedure

1. Stand on top of box with both feet (figure 11.38a).
2. Step off the box, landing on both feet and immediately jumping as high as possible (figure 11.38b).
3. Swing both arms straight up as if making a block or spike (figure 11.38c).
4. Do five jumps.

Key Points

- Don't jump off the box—step off.
- Land on the balls of both feet.
- When landing, flex at the knees to absorb the weight.
- Don't stay on the ground—jump up as quickly as possible.
- Make sure the landing surface is firm yet resilient (carpet or rubber flooring).

Note: To do the box drill routine, you'll need a sturdy box about 12 inches high and a landing surface of at least 18 by 24 inches.

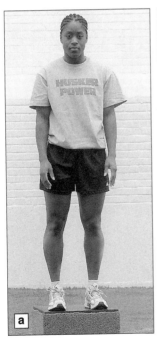 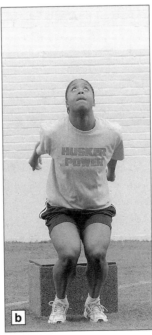 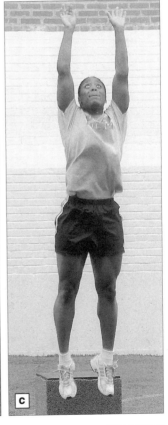

Figure 11.38 Depth jump.

Box Shuffle Step

To develop explosive lateral movements

Procedure

1. Stand to one side of the box with the left foot on the box and the right foot on the ground.
2. Jump up and over the box, the left foot landing on the ground and the right foot on the box.
3. Do this continuously, shuffling back and forth for 20 seconds (see figure 11.39).

Key Point

- Do the drill as quickly as possible with control.

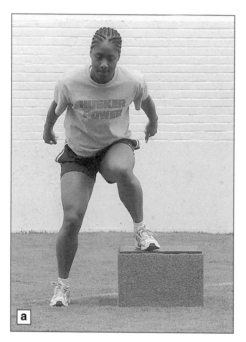 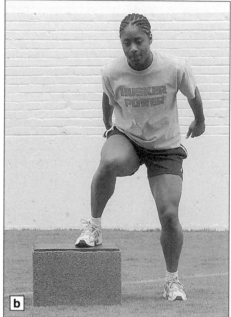

Figure 11.39 Box shuffle step.

Double Box Shuffle Step

To develop explosive lateral movements

Procedure

1. Stand to one side of the box with both feet on the ground.
2. Shuffle onto the box first with the left foot, immediately followed by the right foot.
3. Shuffle off the box first with the left foot, immediately followed by the right foot.
4. Do this continuously, shuffling back and forth for 20 seconds (see figure 11.40).

Key Point

- Do the drill as quickly as possible with control.

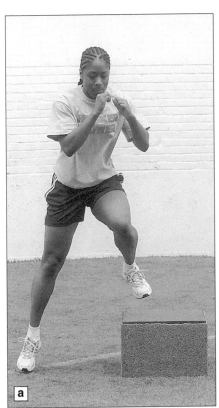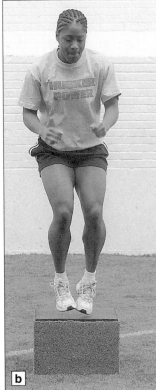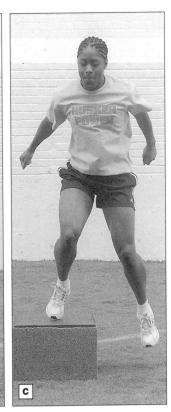

Figure 11.40 Double box shuffle step.

Lateral Box Jumps

To develop explosive lateral movements

Procedure

1. Stand to one side of the box with both feet on the ground.
2. Jump up onto the box with both feet.
3. Jump to the other side of the box with both feet.
4. Do this continuously, jumping back and forth for 20 seconds (see figure 11.41).

Key Point

- Do the drill as quickly as possible with control.

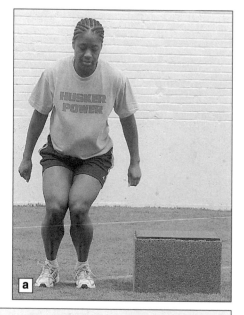

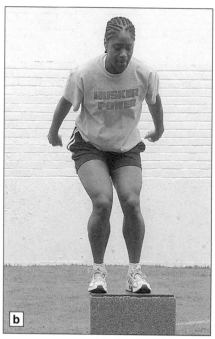

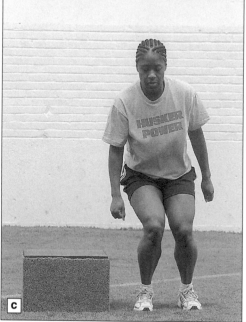

Figure 11.41 Lateral box jump.

This chapter is the meat of this book. Study it carefully. Don't use the metabolic circuit for beginners as it is extremely demanding. Try it with your hardest workers, and they'll see great results that other programs can't match.

12

In-Season and Multisport Programs

Atlanta Braves catcher Bruce Benedict had his best season in the majors in 1983. He recalls, "When I first started in the majors, I just wasn't strong enough physically or mentally." For that reason he would be worn out by late in the season, and his play would suffer. He went on to say, "A couple of years later I wrote the Nebraska strength coach, and he gave me a program of lifting, running, and stretching to follow during the off-season. It really helped me." Consequently, Benedict, 28, played in more games, 135, hit for a better average, .298, had more hits, 130, and more doubles, 15. He was also named to the National League All-Star baseball team for a second time.

A good off-season program is the key to a successful in-season. Don't wait until the season starts to get prepared. Following a good off-season of training, you'll hit your in-season in stride, ready to meet the demands of the challenging weeks ahead.

In-Season

Generally speaking, your goal during the in-season is to train twice a week, always allowing at least one day of rest before a game or contest. You'll want to work all the major muscle groups each week while limiting the number of exercises to as few as possible. This means choosing exercises that work several muscles each. Do squats and bench presses in workout 1 and a choice of cleans along with jammer extensions in workout 2. See table 12.1 for a typical in-season workout schedule. If time allows and the coach wants more work during the season for younger athletes or for athletes who don't play much, the two-day program could become a four-day-per-week program.

Table 12.1 focuses on major exercises and has the repetitions selected that will give the athlete the best opportunity to maintain strength throughout the season. Some coaches will train for maintenance while others might try to improve strength during the season. A good way to determine if the athlete is training too hard during the season is to monitor the vertical jump every two weeks. If you see a big decline, you're overtraining.

Table 12.1 In-Season

Workout 1	Week 1		Week 2		Week 3		Week 4	
Hurdle warm-up	2 × 5		2 × 5		2 × 5		2 × 5	
Snatch squat	2 × 5		2 × 5		2 × 5		2 × 5	
6. Squat	3 × 5		3 × 5		3 × 5		3 × 5	
8a. Bench press	3 × 5		3 × 5		3 × 5		3 × 5	
5. Biceps choice	2 × 10		2 × 10		2 × 10		2 × 10	
11. Push–pull circuit	1 × 10		1 × 10		1 × 10		1 × 10	
Workout 2	**Week 1**		**Week 2**		**Week 3**		**Week 4**	
Hurdle warm-up	2 × 5		2 × 5		2 × 5		2 × 5	
Snatch squat	2 × 5		2 × 5		2 × 5		2 × 5	
*1. Cleans	2 × 5		2 × 5		2 × 5		2 × 5	
3. Jammer extension	2 × 5		2 × 5		2 × 5		2 × 5	
10. Triceps choice	2 × 10		2 × 10		2 × 10		2 × 10	
11. Push–pull circuit	1 × 10		1 × 10		1 × 10		1 × 10	
Date			**Comments**					**INT**
	*Choose from 1a. rack clean, 1b. hang clean, or 1c. power clean.							

Many athletes don't realize that in-season poundages and number of sets should be reduced from what they use during the off-season. One Nebraska athlete lifted a total of 7.5 tons on a typical squat workout during the off-season, whereas his typical in-season workout called for only 2 tons on the squat.

Multisport

The same lifting exercises relate to all power sports. Only one program is necessary to develop explosive power, so if an athlete participates in more than one sport, there's no need to develop specialty programs for the other sports. Improvement in the four performance indicators is the goal for every sport. The characteristics of one sport will have transfer value to others. For example, change of direction and acceleration are basic requirements of every sport. A three-sport athlete doesn't have time to incorporate an off-season during the school year, but it's important that they strength train the entire school year regardless of what sport they're participating in. Ensuring this occurs might require that all involved coaches communicate with each other and agree on the athlete's strength-training program for the year. Because multisport athletes are competing in-season the entire year, they need an in-season program that does more than maintain strength but that doesn't detract from the athlete's performance in contests. This objective can be accomplished through strength training twice a week, once heavy and once easy, with the easy workout coming before the competition. Allow at least one day of no lifting before any competition and at least one day of rest between workouts.

Table 12.2 shows an in-season strength-training program for multisport athletes; here strength and explosive exercises are combined into one workout that's done twice a week. This is different from the traditional in-season program in which the athlete does heavy strength exercises the first workout of the week and explosive lifts for the week's second workout. Multisport athletes don't need a maintenance running program. Participating in the sport takes the place of the running program.

In-season is a time to work on technique and strategy, not overloading the body to gain muscle mass. Touch on each muscle group twice a week during the season to maintain strength.

Table 12.2 Multisport Athlete

Workout 1: Hard	Week 1		Week 2		Week 3		Week 4	
Hurdle warm-up	2 × 5		2 × 5		2 × 5		2 × 5	
Snatch squat	2 × 5		2 × 5		2 × 5		2 × 5	
*1. Cleans	2 × 5		2 × 5		2 × 5		2 × 5	
6. Squat	3 × 5		3 × 5		3 × 5		2 × 5	
8a. Bench press	3 × 5		3 × 5		3 × 5		2 × 5	
Workout 2: Easy	**Week 1**		**Week 2**		**Week 3**		**Week 4**	
Hurdle warm-up	2 × 5		2 × 5		2 × 5		2 × 5	
Snatch squat	2 × 5		2 × 5		2 × 5		2 × 5	
*1. Cleans	2 × 5		2 × 5		2 × 5		2 × 5	
6. Squat	2 × 5		2 × 5		2 × 5		2 × 5	
8a. Bench press	2 × 5		2 × 5		2 × 5		2 × 5	
Date	**Comments**							**INT**
	*Choose from 1a. rack clean, 1b. hang clean, or 1c. power clean.							

5 Championships Might Have Been 10

In-season conditioning was a major factor during the 1995 Orange Bowl win over a fatigued Miami. In most cases, it is the work in the off-season that leads to success in-season. A little more work in the 1981 summer off-season program might have paid dividends when the Huskers needed only 50 yards at the end of the game to win and couldn't get a first down. In-season strength and conditioning showed in the 1998 Orange Bowl win over Tennessee. Scott Frost, the most physical quarterback in Nebraska history, still holds the strength index record for quarterbacks based on his squat and hang clean index points. Read about ten games in which Nebraska had a chance to win a national championship ring.

1971 Orange Bowl. Nebraska won its first national championship 17–12 with a win over the LSU Tigers. The Tigers led 12–10 going into the fourth quarter. A 13-play drive in the fourth quarter ended with quarterback Jerry Tagge crossing the goal line to take the lead. Texas and Ohio State had been ranked higher than us, but both teams lost their bowl games earlier that day, so everything fell into place for Nebraska to be number one. This was an exciting time for a young strength coach doing graduate work.

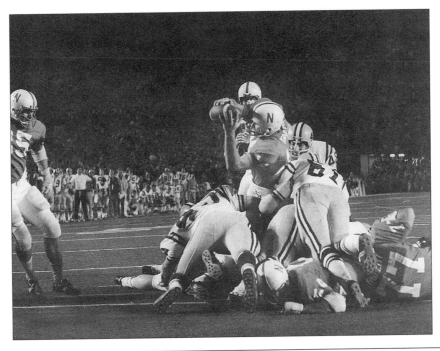

Quarterback Jerry Tagge powers over the goal line to give Nebraska its first national championship in the 1971 Orange Bowl.

1972 Orange Bowl. One of the most memorable football games occurred in 1971 as Nebraska beat Oklahoma 35–31. Nebraska captured the win following a long drive in the final eight minutes. Jerry Tagge handed off to Jeff Kinney on every play but one, a desperation third-down pass to Johnny Rodgers, who made a diving catch to keep the drive alive. Behind a tough offensive line, Kinney plunged over the goal line from the three for the win. The game of the century was played in Norman, Oklahoma, for the Big Eight title and sent Nebraska to the Orange Bowl for a national title match with Alabama. Nebraska beat Alabama 38–6.

(continued)

(continued)

1982 Orange Bowl. The Clemson Tigers defeated Nebraska 22–15. William "Refrigerator" Perry and the Tiger defense allowed Nebraska only 8 points in the fourth quarter. We had only 50 yards to drive for the win and couldn't get it done. As a result, top ranked Clemson won its first national title.

1984 Orange Bowl. Miami beat the Huskers 31–30. We scored two touchdowns in the fourth quarter with less than five minutes remaining. On fourth down and 28 yards to go to the end zone, Jeff Smith took a pitch from Turner Gill and ran into pay dirt. An extra point and tie would have given Coach Osborne the national title, but he made the gutsy choice and went for the 2-point conversion. The ball fell to the ground incomplete as Turner Gill's pass was tipped, and Miami won its first national title. Osborne gained national recognition for going for the win instead of the tie.

1994 Orange Bowl. Nebraska had taken the lead with 1:16 left on the clock, but we let a national championship slip away as Florida State kicked a field goal with 21 seconds left and won its first title with an 18–16 win. That summer, I asked Randy Gobel to put 1:16 on the scoreboard in the Nebraska stadium every day along with the words "Unfinished Business." No one had ever used the scoreboard in summer training before. I asked the players to do 1 minute and 16 seconds of additional conditioning each day as a reminder that 1:16 was on the clock in the Orange Bowl against Florida State when Nebraska let them get back into the game. This reminder became a rallying point in the fourth quarter of several games during the 1994 season. In the fourth quarter of each game, our players displayed an extra burst of will power. They were determined not to lose, and they knew they had prepared not to lose. The extra work they did in the summer wasn't much—in fact, it wasn't even a continuous 1:16 seconds of work. They ran through a row of hurdles, which took about five seconds, then stood in line until their turn to run back. But the extra work had an amazing impact throughout the season.

1995 Orange Bowl. Nebraska won 24–17 over Miami, scoring two touchdowns in the fourth quarter. The extra work we did in the summer was evident. Miami supposedly had more talented athletes, but fatigue became a factor for them in the fourth quarter, allowing us to score two touchdowns on fullback Cory Schlesinger's runs up the middle. The Nebraska defense stopped Miami three plays and out for seven series in a row at the end of the game. This was the best example I've ever seen of how conditioning can affect a game. Miami was exhausted, and Nebraska got stronger as the game went into the fourth quarter. Miami had been running longer runs to prepare for the Orange Bowl. They must not have realized they were training the wrong energy system. Nebraska football coaches did a great job of keeping the game close enough for their plan to work in the fourth quarter. Our team motto that year had been "Unfinished Business." After our huge win in the Orange Bowl, the sports information office created a poster and video titled "Finished Business."

1996 Fiesta Bowl. Nebraska won 62–24 over Florida with an NCAA bowl record 524 yards rushing. Coach Ron Zook, now the head coach of Florida, was a special teams coach for Florida at the time of the national championship game at the Fiesta Bowl. Ron and I were talking on the field just before the game. "Boy, your guys are big," he commented as he watched the two teams warm up. I told him, "The big guys aren't out here yet." I explained the team came out in three groups, and only two of the groups were on the field so far, the receivers and the backs. The big linemen hadn't come out yet. Just then, about 30 linemen came running out onto the field from the north end zone. Zook's face turned pale as he saw how big the Nebraska linemen were. We finished the year with our most impressive victory in that national championship game. Florida didn't know what hit them. Our team's motto that year was "Leave no doubt," and the 62–24 drubbing did just that. Jerry Schmidt, strength coach for Florida before moving to Oklahoma, spoke to me at halftime when Nebraska was up 35–10. As the two teams were walking to the locker room, he told me, "You guys are good."

1996 Big-12 championship. Nebraska had won back-to-back national titles, and in January we got together for the start of the winter program. I explained to our players that Alabama and Oklahoma were the only other schools ever to have been in our position, with an opportunity to win three straight. After winning in 1964 and 1965, Alabama went undefeated in 1966 but was not awarded the national championship. They finished third behind Notre Dame and Michigan State, who tied 10–10. Ara Parseghian was criticized for going for the tie rather than the win, but doing so meant Notre Dame was named national champion. But Alabama came the closest any team had ever come to winning three straight.

I had wanted to accomplish this for many years, and now we were in position to make it happen. I had T-shirts printed for the players and

(continued)

(continued)

asked a local artist to draw a player's hand. No words appeared on the drawing, just the image of three taped fingers.

The Big 12 conference was formed in 1996, and a Big 12 conference playoff game was scheduled for the first time for December 7th. Coach Osborne was the only head coach in the conference who did not favor a playoff game. He knew that a playoff game might eliminate one of the major teams in the conference from a national championship game, and sure enough that's exactly what happened in the very first year. Nebraska breezed through the conference North Division 8–0 and entered the championship game 10–1, whereas Texas was 7–4 and representing the South Division. Nebraska was favored to beat Texas, which would set up a national championship game with Florida State. Wow, what a great opportunity Nebraska had. We had beaten Miami, and then Florida, and now we would have a chance to beat Florida State. The stage would be set for three straight national championships, which had never happened before. It would be Nebraska against the entire state of Florida. It would be revenge against Florida State for the 21 seconds left on the clock when they pulled ahead to win at the end of the 1993 season. But it wasn't to be. All these things came to an end with a fourth-down pass play by a gutsy Texas team. Leading Nebraska 30–27 with 2:40 left and the ball sitting at its own 28-yard line, Texas made one of the most courageous fourth-down and inches plays in college football history. "If you're going to be a champion, you have to go for it. You have to seize the day," head coach John Mackovic said later. With the clock rolling and no timeout called, quarterback James Brown quickly stepped under center and received the ball immediately. Brown was prepared to run after faking a handoff to Priest Holmes and pivoting to his left. But the junior signal caller stunned everyone when he stopped and lofted a pass downfield to a wide-open Derek Lewis for what turned into a 61-yard completion. That play, later voted college football's play of the year, set up Priest Holmes' touchdown run and allowed the three-touchdown underdogs to claim their first-ever Big-12 championship with a 37–27 victory.

1998 Orange Bowl. Nebraska won 42–17 over Tennessee, as the Osborne era came to an end with three national titles in four years. Leading 14–3 at halftime, the Huskers showed their dominance, scoring on all three of their third-quarter possessions. Scott Frost put on a show at quarterback, and Ahman Green put the game out of reach as he rushed for an Orange Bowl-record 206 yards and two touchdowns. The Nebraska defense held Peyton Manning to a season-low 134 yards in the air and forced three turnovers.

2002 Rose Bowl. Miami won the BCS national championship easily, 37–14. The Rose Bowl was basically over in the first quarter. Eric Crouch moved the ball to the 49-yard line but fumbled. The next play, Miami threw a deep pass to Andre Johnson for a 49-yard touchdown. The Nebraska defender had been pulled to the ground, leaving the receiver completely alone. No penalty was called, and Miami scored effortlessly. Miami kicked off after the score, and Nebraska fumbled the ball, setting Miami up again. The Hurricanes marched 86 yards in 5 plays to go up 14–0. Nebraska scored 14 in the fourth quarter, but it was too little too late. A few days after the poor showing in the Rose Bowl, I was in the St. Louis airport, and a woman walking the same direction noticed an N on my shirt and commented, "Aren't you embarrassed to wear that shirt?" I'm sure I looked puzzled by the comment and wasn't quite sure how to respond, but I managed to say, "I have never been embarrassed to be associated with Nebraska in 30 years." She just walked off without further comment, but I wish I could have talked with her more to learn what could have caused her to make a comment like that.

No team wins every game, but Nebraska won more that any other school during the 34-year span that I was involved with them as a strength coach. The problem is that in our what-have-you-done-lately society, if you're not *the* winner in a particular year, then you're a loser. Only two football teams are allowed to compete for the title, and one of them is going to lose. I guess that makes them a loser. But what does that mean for all the other teams that didn't have a good enough record to participate in the final game? Are they also losers? Somehow we need to appreciate a high level of achievement and dispose of the loser label.

13

Anaerobic, Speed, and Agility Training

For many years I believed an aerobic base was necessary before starting speed and agility drills. But research by Dr. Michael Stone convinced me to skip the distance running and incorporate anaerobic interval training. The first year Nebraska linemen discontinued distance running, they gained an average of 30 pounds during the summer program. We found that any running takes away from the recovery ability for strength gains from lifting and concluded it takes only about four weeks to condition for a power sport. Most coaches want to run more than Nebraska strength coaches would recommend. A good rule of thumb is "No running during the base lifting phase." Focus all efforts on weight room recovery during the base phase.

Interval Running

The best way to set up a running program is to follow interval training principles. The drills are short bursts of speed or agility drills followed by a rest interval. Rather than having all your athletes run together at the same time, it works best to build rest into the drill. While two or three athletes run, the others are in line preparing to run or are returning to the back of the line for their next run.

Each drill has a prescribed rest interval based on the energy needs of the sport. As reported in chapter 4, football has a work-to-rest ratio of 1 to 10. That means if the drill lasts 5 seconds, the rest period should be 50 seconds. To increase the intensity of the drill, have your athletes race each other or time them as they're doing the drill.

Build a two-minute rest period between sets of drills for power sports. A common training error is to make the rest interval too short. I've seen coaches make their athletes run from one station to the next with little or no rest between drills. This makes athletes pace themselves to get through the workout, which means less intensity during the drills. Athletes should be giving their best effort each time it's their turn, which means giving them adequate rest between drills and between sets of drills. Work water breaks into rest periods to ensure proper hydration.

Study the "Big Picture" in chapter 10 to gradually introduce speed followed by agility drills. Begin with lifting four days a week with no running for a few weeks. Add speed drills to the program twice a week. Eventually add agility drills so that athletes are running four days per week.

Conditioning Warm-Up Drills

1. High knees—10 yards
2. Heel-ups—10 yards
3. High knees with foreleg extension—20 yards
4. Carioca drill—20 yards
5. Build-ups

High Knees—10 Yards

To develop muscles needed for a fast long stride and flexibility in the hamstrings. All good sprinters have a good high-knee action. The higher the knee-lift while running, the longer the stride.

Procedure

1. Drive knees high and forcefully (figure 13.1).
2. When you lift one leg, the other leg should be fully extended.
3. Bend forward slightly at the waist while keeping the back straight.
4. Drive elbows vigorously.
5. Relax face and arms.
6. Take short, quick steps.

Key Points

- Avoid leaning back or taking long steps.
- Maintain proper forward lean.
- Make sure thighs become parallel to the ground.
- Arms should swing freely at the shoulders with good arm action.
- Keep your face and neck relaxed.
- Achieve at least 30 steps in 10 yards.

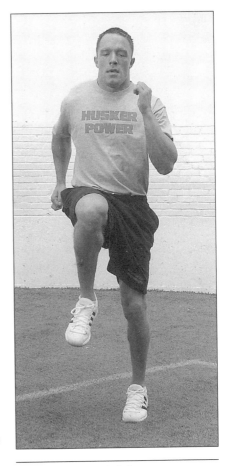

Figure 13.1 High knees.

Heel-Ups—10 Yards

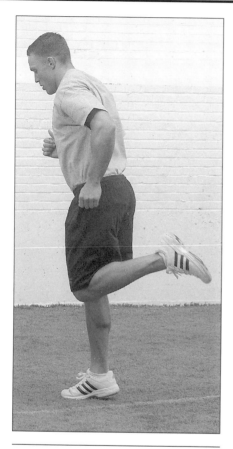

Figure 13.2 Heel-ups.

To develop strength in the hamstrings and flexibility in the thighs. When the heels come up to the hips while running, the thighs swing through faster, which increases stride frequency.

Procedure

1. Alternately swing heel of each foot up to the buttocks (figure 13.2).
2. Action is quick, with a smooth swinging motion produced at the knee joint.

Key Points

- Maintain good forward lean.
- Keep knees pointed down toward the ground.
- Heels should swing freely at the knees.
- Heels should come in contact with the hips.
- Stay on your toes.
- Arms hang relaxed at sides.
- Avoid moving forward too fast, using the arms, or lifting the knees by flexing at the hips.

High Knees With Foreleg Extension—20 Yards

To develop flexibility in the hamstrings and increase ability to reach with foreleg

Procedure

1. Lift left knee high.
2. When left knee reaches highest position, the right leg does a little skip.
3. As you skip, extend the left foreleg until it's parallel to the ground (figure 13.3).
4. Repeat on the other side.

Key Points

- Maintain proper forward lean.
- Thigh should become parallel to the floor before knee is straightened.
- The foreleg should extend out and up forcefully.
- Avoid incomplete extension of the foreleg.
- Movement should be rhythmic.

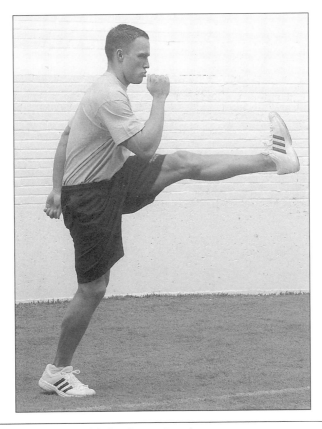

Figure 13.3 High knees with foreleg extension.

Carioca Drill—20 Yards

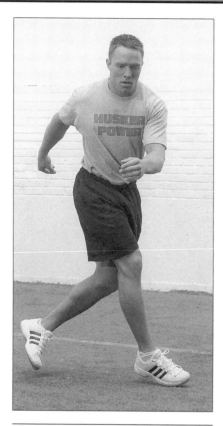

Figure 13.4 Carioca drill.

To develop mobility and balance

Procedure

1. Get into a power stance with knees flexed and shoulders facing squarely forward.
2. Move laterally to your left, crossing the right foot over in front of the left (figure 13.4), then bringing the right foot behind on the next step.
3. If moving right, reverse the procedure.
4. While moving, remain in your power stance. Keep shoulders square and get good hip rotation.

Key Points

- Start from a power stance.
- Twist hips around as far as possible.
- Keep shoulders square, not twisting with the hips.
- Take the biggest steps possible.
- Maintain the power position throughout.
- Don't move too fast or you will lose your hip rotation.

Build-Ups

To improve acceleration

Procedure

1. Start off with a standing start and go into a slow run.
2. Gradually build up speed, reaching full speed at 40 yards.
3. Once full speed is achieved at 40 yards, gradually slow down over the final 20 yards. See figure 13.5.

Key Points

- Don't accelerate too fast.
- Be running at full speed at 40 yards.
- Avoid running at full speed after 40 yards.
- Use good sprinting form.

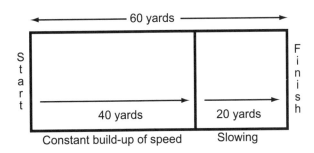

Figure 13.5   Build-ups.

Speed Drills

Schedule heavy legwork after running speed drills rather than before.

Weeks 1–2	Number of times
Build-ups (40 yards)	4
Form starts	4
Position starts	4
Flying 10s	2
Power skips (height)	2
Power skips (distance)	2

Weeks 3–4	Number of times
Build-ups (40 yards)	4
Form starts	4
Position starts	4
Flying 20s	2
Power skips (height)	2
Power skips (distance)	2
Harness routine	1
Weeks 5–6	
Build-ups (40 yards)	4
Form starts	4
Position starts	4
Flying 30s	2
Bag jumps	4
Harness routine	1
Weeks 7–8	
Build-ups (40 yards)	4
Form starts	4
Position starts	4
Hollow sprints	4
Bag jumps	4
Harness routine	2

Build-Ups (40 yards)

To improve acceleration

Procedure

1. From a standing position, move into a slow run.
2. Gradually build up speed until reaching full speed at 40 yards.
3. Once full speed is achieved at 40 yards, gradually slow down over the final 20 yards.

Key Points

- Don't accelerate too fast.
- Reach full speed at 40 yards.

Form Starts

To develop good stance

Procedure

1. Front foot is 3 to 6 inches behind starting line.
2. Place the fingers of the hand opposite the front foot directly on the starting line with thumb and forefinger parallel to the line.
3. The other hand is at the hip of the forward leg; the elbow is pointed up (see figure 13.6).
4. The back foot is 6 to 12 inches behind the heel of the forward foot and 2 to 4 inches to the side.
5. The hips should be slightly above shoulder height.
6. The shoulders should be slightly ahead of the starting line with most of the body weight on the front leg and hand.
7. Keep eyes focused 2 to 3 feet in front of the starting line.

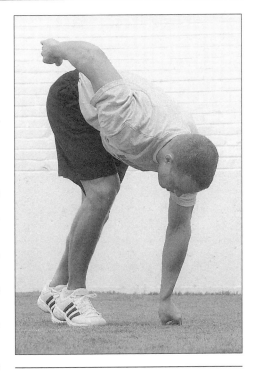

Figure 13.6   Form starts.

Key Points

- Make sure hips are higher than the shoulders.
- Don't let arm rest on front leg.

Position Starts

To develop good acceleration from the player's starting stance

Procedure

1. Assume on-the-field starting stance.
2. On coach's command, explode out of the starting stance for the required distance.

Key Points

- Get good explosion out of the stance.
- Make sure the first step is forward.

Flying 10s

To improve acceleration and stride frequency

Procedure

1. Start running at half-speed, building speed at each stride for the first 30 yards.
2. Acceleration should be continuous for the first 30 yards.
3. When you reach the 30-yard mark, be running at full speed.
4. Continue to sprint for 10 more yards. See figure 13.7.

Key Points

- Don't accelerate too fast; the build-up should be constant for 30 yards.
- Sprint the entire final 10 yards.

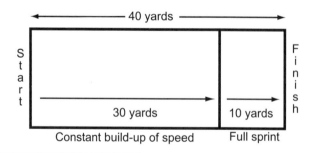

Figure 13.7 Flying 10s.

Flying 20s

To improve acceleration and stride frequency

Procedure

1. Start running at half-speed, building speed at each stride for the first 30 yards.
2. Acceleration should be continuous for the first 30 yards.
3. At the 30-yard mark, be running at full speed.
4. Continue to sprint for 20 more yards. See figure 13.8.

Key Points

- Don't accelerate too fast; the build-up should be constant for 30 yards.
- Sprint the entire final 20 yards.

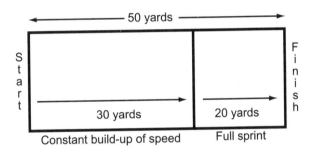

Figure 13.8 Flying 20s.

Power Skips for Height

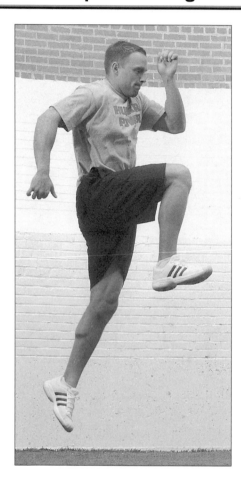

To increase explosion in the legs and hips

Procedure

1. Begin skipping, pushing off explosively with the back leg.
2. Opposite leg drives knee up as high as possible, trying to achieve maximal height (figure 13.9).
3. Prepare for contact with the ground; repeat with opposite leg immediately upon landing.

Key Points

- Skip as high as possible with triple extension of the back leg.
- Drive knee to chest.

Figure 13.9 Power skips for height.

Power Skips for Distance

To increase explosion in the legs and hips

Procedure

1. Begin skipping, pushing off explosively with the back leg.
2. Opposite leg drives knee up and out as high as possible. Try to achieve maximal distance (see figure 13.10).
3. Prepare for contact with the ground and repeat with opposite leg immediately upon landing.

Key Points

- Skip as far as possible with triple extension of the back leg.
- Drive knee up and out.

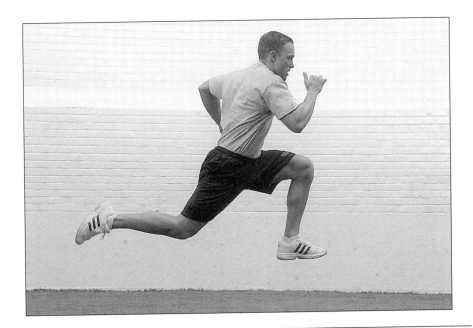

Figure 13.10   Power skips for distance.

Harness Routine

To develop acceleration and get to top speed quickly

Procedure

1. Find an area with 50 to 60 yards of flat running surface.
2. Drive off the hind leg extending completely at ankles, knees, and hips.
3. Forward leg carries to high-knee position.
4. Hold arms at a 90-degree angle.
5. On the backswing, drive elbows back and up.
6. On the forward swing, bring hands level with the shoulders.
7. Maintain a good forward lean.
8. Focus eyes 20 to 30 yards in front.
9. One rep includes a 10-yard run down and back forward (figure 13.11a), down and back shuffle (figure 13.11b), and down and back with backpedal (figure 13.11c).

Key Points

- Pump arms quickly with good form.
- Apply proper resistance.
- Maintain correct body lean and running form.
- Drive up knees and heels.

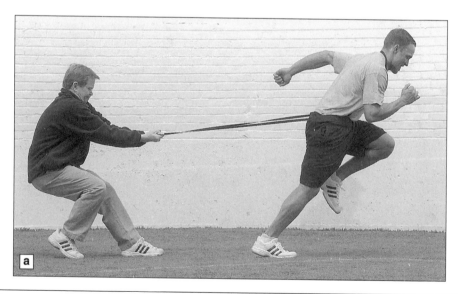

Figure 13.11 Harness routine: *(a)* Forward, *(b)* back shuffle, *(c)* backpedal.

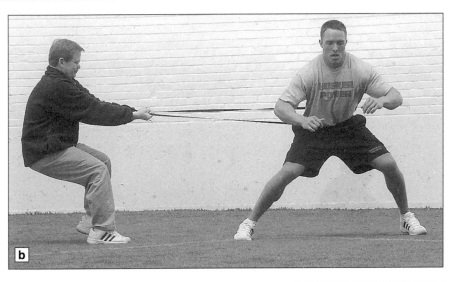

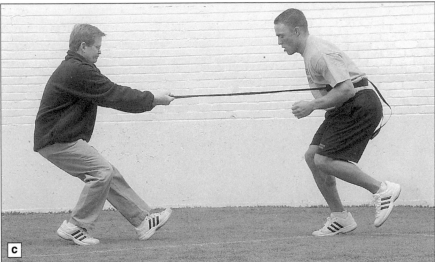

Figure 13.11 *(continued)*

Flying 30s

To improve acceleration and stride frequency

Procedure

1. Start running at half-speed, building speed at each stride for the first 30 yards.
2. Acceleration should be continuous for the first 30 yards.
3. Attain full speed at the 30-yard mark.
4. Continue to sprint for 30 more yards. See figure 13.12.

Key Points

- Don't accelerate too fast; the build-up should be constant for 30 yards.
- Sprint the entire second 30 yards.

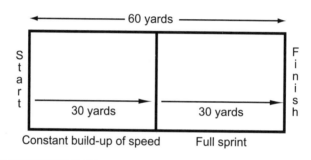

Figure 13.12 Flying 30s.

Bag Jumps

To develop explosiveness and acceleration

Procedure

1. Stand facing a series of bags stacked two high. Begin by jumping over the first set of bags.
2. Assist the jump by moving arms explosively and bringing knees to chest (see figure 13.13).
3. After contact with ground, quickly jump over second set of bags.
4. Continue through all sets of bags.

Key Points

- Jump quickly—don't spend much time on the ground.
- Use your arms to help jump over the bags.
- Don't stutter-step between the bags.
- Bring feet over the bags, not out around the sides.

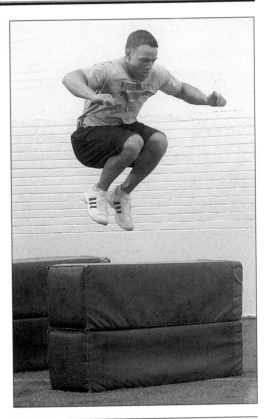

Figure 13.13 Bag jumps.

Hollow Sprints

To improve acceleration

Procedure
1. Run at half speed for 20 yards.
2. Sprint at full speed for 20 yards.
3. Slow back to the original half speed and run another 20 yards.
4. Sprint at full speed for 20 yards.
5. Run at half speed the last 20 yards. See figure 13.14.

Key Points
- Change from half speed to full speed at designated points.
- Accelerate to full intensity at top speed.
- Sprint at full speed for the required distance.

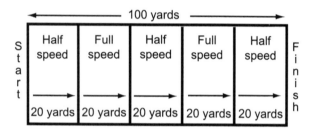

Figure 13.14 Hollow sprints.

Agility Drills

Start agility drills in week five. (The first four weeks are speed drills only.)

Weeks 5–6	Number of times
Rope routine	1
Bag routine	1
Jump rope routine	1
Pro agility	4
Nebraska agility	4
Three-corner drill	4
Sprint ladder	4

Weeks 7–8	Number of times
Rope routine	1
Bag routine	1
Jump rope routine	1
Pro agility	4
Nebraska agility	4
Three-corner drill	4
Sprint ladder	2
Shuffle ladder	2
Backpedal ladder	2

Rope Routine: Every Hole

To develop high-knee action, peripheral vision, and footwork

Procedure

1. Run forward using high-knee action.
2. Right foot hits every hole on right side; left foot hits every hole on left side (figure 13.15).
3. Use good arm action.

Key Points

- Lift knees high.
- Pump arms.
- Use quick feet.
- Keep head up and eyes focused straight ahead.

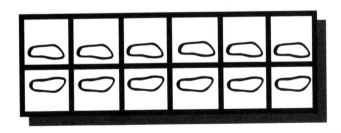

Figure 13.15 Every-hole rope routine.

Rope Routine: Every Other Hole

To develop high-knee action, peripheral vision, flexibility, and footwork

Procedure

1. Run forward using high-knee action with a slight forward lean.
2. Right foot hits every other hole on right side; left foot hits every other hole on left side (figure 13.16).
3. Use good arm action.

Key Points

- Lift knees high.
- Pump arms.
- Be quick.
- Don't lean backward.
- Keep head up and eyes focused straight ahead.

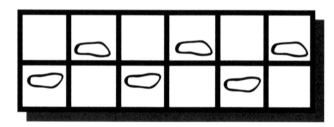

Figure 13.16 Every-other-hole rope routine.

Rope Routine: Lateral Step

To develop foot quickness, flexibility, and peripheral vision

Procedure

1. Run laterally using high-knee action and hitting every hole (see figure 13.17).

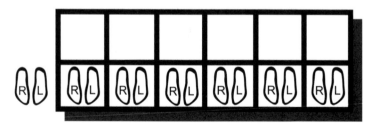

Figure 13.17 Lateral-step rope routine.

2. Use only one side of the ropes.
3. Go one direction leading with the right foot; go the other direction leading with the left foot.

Key Points
- Keep shoulders and hips square.
- Keep head up and eyes focused straight ahead.
- Be quick.

Bag Routine: **Change of Direction**

To develop quick foot action, flexibility, and high-knee action

Procedure
1. Start at either the right or left side at one end of the bags.
2. Run forward toward the other side of the bag.
3. Planting the outside foot at the end of the bag, explode forward toward the other end of the next bag (see figure 13.18).

Key Points
- Push off with the outside foot.
- Maintain good acceleration through the bags.

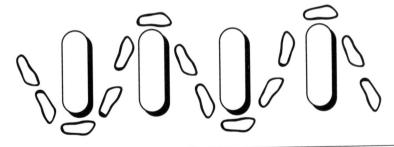

Figure 13.18   Change-of-direction bag routine.

Bag Routine: Shuffle

To develop foot coordination, quickness, strength, and flexibility in the abductors and adductors

Procedure

1. Start at either the right or left side at one end of the bags facing the row of bags.
2. Shuffle diagonally beyond the first bag.
3. Change directions and shuffle diagonally to the end of the second bag.
4. Continue shuffling through the bags. See figure 13.19.

Key Points

- Stay low throughout the drill.
- Don't cross your feet.
- Push off with the trailing foot.
- Push off with the outside foot when changing direction.

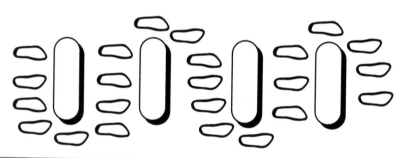

Figure 13.19 Shuffle bag routine.

Bag Routine: Forward and Backpedal

To develop quick foot action, flexibility, and high-knee action

Procedure

1. Assume a two-point stance with knees slightly bent, torso upright, head up, and hands and arms away from body. On command, run forward to the end of the bag.
2. Backpedal through to the other end, then forward.
3. Repeat through all the bags, ending with a five-yard sprint forward. See figure 13.20.

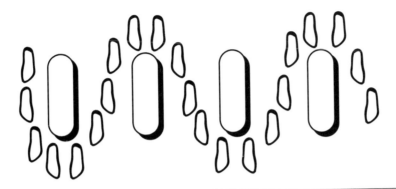

Figure 13.20 Forward-and-backpedal bag routine.

Key Points
- Stay low throughout the drill.
- Keep weight forward during the backpedal.
- Avoid false steps when changing directions.

Jump Rope Routine: Single Bunny Hop

To develop timing, agility, balance, and leg strength

Procedure
1. Stand with feet near a yard line at the sideline.
2. Jump back and forth over the line with one foot as you move forward (figure 13.21).
3. Switch feet at the halfway point without stopping.

Key Points
- Stay as close to the line as possible.
- Keep eyes and head up.
- You can also do this drill jumping backward.

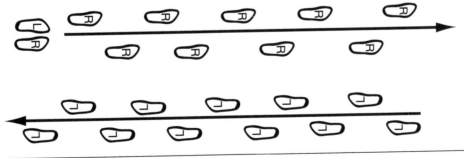

Figure 13.21 Single bunny hop rope routine.

Jump Rope Routine: Double Bunny Hop

To develop timing, agility, and balance

Procedure

1. Stand with feet near a yard line at the sideline.
2. Jump back and forth over the line as you move forward (see figure 13.22).

Key Points

- Keep feet close together.
- Stay as close to the line as possible.
- Keep eyes and head up.
- Use quick foot action.
- You can also do this drill jumping backward.

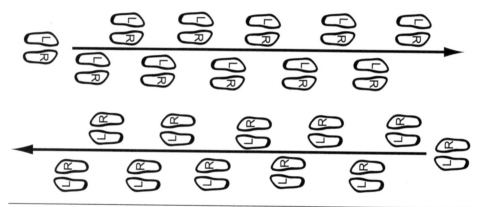

Figure 13.22 Double bunny hop rope routine.

Jump Rope Routine: Scissors

To develop timing, agility, balance, and lateral movement

Procedure

1. Stand at the sideline with feet straddling the yard line.
2. Scissors-step down the line and back (figure 13.23).

Key Points

- Stay on the line as you move forward.
- Keep eyes and head up.
- Each foot stays on its own side of the line.

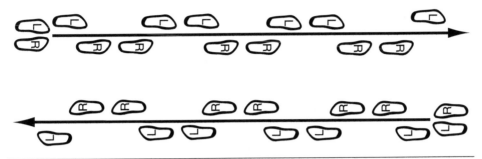

Figure 13.23   Scissors rope routine.

Jump Rope Routine: Ali Shuffle

To develop timing, agility, balance, and coordination

Procedure

1. Stand at the sideline with feet to one side of the yard line.
2. Do the Ali shuffle as you move laterally down the line. (One foot goes forward of the line, and the other foot stays behind the line. Switch feet as you jump into the air to the front and back of the line). See figure 13.24.

Key Points

- Go to the front and back of the line as you switch feet.
- Keep eyes and head up.
- Go both to the right and left.

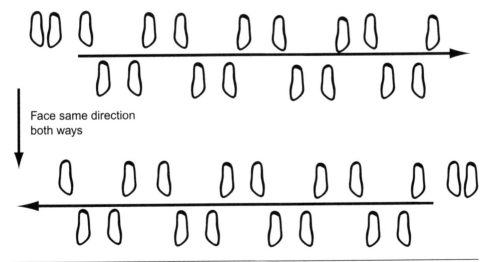

Face same direction both ways

Figure 13.24   Ali-shuffle rope routine.

Pro Agility Drill

To improve footwork, change of direction, and reaction time

Procedure

1. From a two-point stance, straddle the middle line.
2. Sprint to the left line and touch it with the left hand.
3. Push off forcefully and sprint back across the middle line to the right line and touch that line with your right hand.
4. Sprint back to the left, finishing at the middle line. See figure 13.25.

Key Points

- When running to the right, always touch the line with the right hand; when running to the left, always touch the line with the left hand. This ensures that you push off with the opposite feet.
- Be sure to touch the line with your hand.
- Stay low when changing directions.
- You can have up to five athletes do the drill at the same time and race each other.
- A coach can stand in front and point to the right or left to start the athletes.

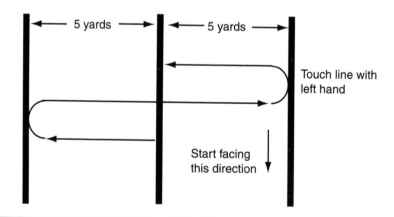

Figure 13.25 Pro agility drill.

Nebraska Agility Drill

To improve foot quickness and change of direction

Procedure

1. Start in a three-point stance on the first line.
2. Sprint to the first cone and make a right turn.
3. Return to the starting line. Go around the second cone with a left turn.
4. Run to the five-yard line and touch it with your fingers, then backpedal across the starting line to the finish. See figure 13.26.

Key Points

- Don't knock the cones over.
- Be sure to touch the line with your hand.
- Stay low on the backpedal.
- Keep feet moving around the cone as quickly as possible while staying low.

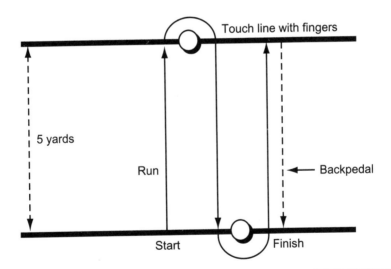

Figure 13.26 Nebraska agility drill.

Three-Corner Drill

To improve footwork, change of direction, acceleration, and deceleration

Procedure

1. Start in a three-point stance on the first line.
2. Sprint to the first cone, plant your left foot and drive off it, shuffling right to the second cone.
3. At the second cone, backpedal to the third cone.
4. At the third cone, plant the left foot and break at a 45-degree angle. See figure 13.27.

Key Points

- Have good acceleration while sprinting to the first cone.
- Don't cross the legs on the shuffle step.
- Stay low on the backpedal.
- Maintain good acceleration after the third cone.
- Keep eyes up; don't look for cones.

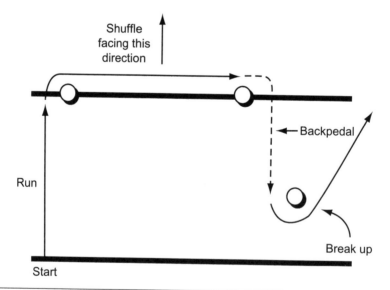

Figure 13.27 Three-corner drill.

Sprint Ladder

To develop agility and conditioning

Procedure

1. Begin in a three-point stance on the start line.
2. Sprint 5 yards to the first line and touch it with your right foot; return to the starting line and touch it with your left foot.
3. Sprint 10 yards to the second line and touch it with your right foot; return to the starting line and touch it with your left foot.
4. Sprint 5 yards to the first line and touch it with your right foot; return to the starting line. See figure 13.28.

Key Points

- Touch the line at 5-yard intervals with the right foot and the starting line with the left foot (push off with each leg, and don't run in circles).
- Run all runs at full speed.

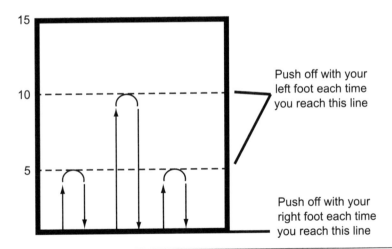

Figure 13.28   Sprint ladder.

Shuffle Ladder

To develop agility, conditioning, strength, and flexibility in the abductor and adductors

Procedure

1. Begin in a two-point stance perpendicular to the start line.
2. Shuffle 5 yards to the first line and touch it with your right foot; shuffle to the starting line and touch it with your left foot.
3. Shuffle 10 yards to the second line and touch it with your right foot; shuffle to the starting line and touch it with your left foot.
4. Shuffle 5 yards to the first line and touch it with your right foot; shuffle to the starting line. See figure 13.29.

Key Points

- Touch the line at 5-yard intervals with the right foot and the starting line with the left foot (push off with each leg, and don't run in circles).
- Don't cross your feet.
- Keep back straight while staying low.
- The coach should stand so the athletes are always facing him or her.

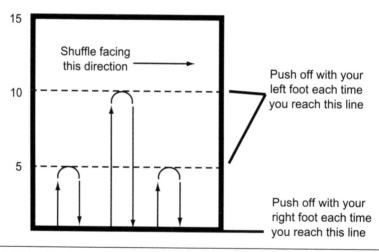

Figure 13.29   Shuffle ladder.

Backpedal Ladder

To develop agility, conditioning, and change of direction

Procedure

1. Begin in a two-point stance standing with your back to the start line.
2. Backpedal 5 yards to the first line, touch the line with either foot; sprint to the start line and touch it with either foot.
3. Backpedal 10 yards to the second line and touch it with either foot; sprint to the start line and touch it with either foot.
4. Backpedal 5 yards to the first line and touch it with either foot; sprint back to the start line. See figure 13.30.

Key Points

- Keep low on the backpedal.
- Run all runs at full speed.
- Maintain good acceleration coming out of the backpedal.

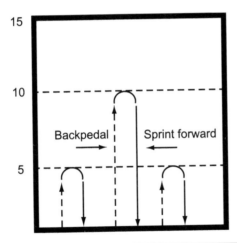

Figure 13.30   Backpedal ladder.

I have given thousands of clinics over the years and have had the opportunity to meet with thousands of high school coaches. Most have the lifting principles worked into their programs and do a pretty good job in the lifting area. The one area in which coaches need a little more work is buying into anaerobic training. Coach Osborne, who is a jogger, bought into the concept, and his teams were almost unbeatable. Many coaches want to run athletes aerobically. This is not necessary. Most coaches work with power sports that require a rest interval between drills. If athletes don't get enough rest, they will pace themselves and not have the intensity that is needed on each drill. Too much running can also drain away the strength gains you're looking for and cause injuries.

14

Future Developments in Sports Conditioning

Strength training has undoubtedly made competitive athletics more explosive and more exciting; athletes have made great improvements in strength, power, and speed under the supervision of specialized strength and conditioning coaches.

On the collegiate level, where strength and conditioning coaches were first introduced, these coaches have become an integral part of the coaching staff. A large portion of the athletes' time is spent under the direction of the head strength and conditioning coach and his or her staff. In fact, in most cases, no other member of the athletic department has more personal contact with the athlete than the strength and conditioning coach does. Whereas position coaches work with a set group of athletes, most strength and conditioning coaches work with entire teams. This typically makes for a good rapport between the strength and conditioning coach and the athletes; many athletes seek advice regarding nutrition, supplementation, conditioning, general health and fitness, and more from their strength and conditioning coach.

The strength and conditioning coach must be highly trained in many physiological principles, such as energy systems, neuromuscular development, and cardiorespiratory fitness, and also be able to motivate and train athletes effectively. To become certified, a strength and conditioning coach needs at least a bachelor's degree, and many have their masters or doctorate degrees. This is not a job just anyone can do. These coaches are highly trained and committed to helping their athletes safely reach their full athletic potential through maximizing strength, power, and speed, while reducing risk of injury. The strength coach is a valuable key to the future of sport in America.

How the NSCA Was Formed

The community of strength coaches wasn't always as organized as it is now, as I found out during a chance conversation with Boyd McWhirter, commissioner of the Southeastern Conference (SEC). Our dialogue before the 1977 Nebraska–Alabama football game planted the first seed in my mind of the need for strength coaches to become identified as professionals within university athletic departments. On explaining my role as strength coach at Nebraska to McWhirter, who was until then unaware that such a position existed, he asked whether any strength coaches were employed in the SEC. Alerted to the ignorance of the value of strength coaches and strength training, I set out to identify as many strength coaches as possible through a mass-mailing questionnaire, and then I compiled a national strength coaches directory. A $5 donation was requested from each "subscriber" to fund the directory's February 22, 1978, publication.

Not long thereafter, Pete Martinelli, then of the University of New Mexico and later of Oklahoma, and Jim Williams, my first assistant, then of Wyoming and later of the Philadelphia Eagles, New York Jets, and New York Giants, suggested to me that I form an association for strength coaches. At the time, those in the profession were largely isolated from one another with little opportunity to share strength-training ideas. An association would offer college strength coaches a fraternity in which they could communicate with like-minded professionals.

In 1978, Bill Starr included the following short passage in his book *The Strongest Shall Survive:* "The future holds great promise for those of us in the profession of making athletes stronger. We must, in the next few years, have some avenue whereby we can exchange training ideas and new training concepts. We ideally should come together periodically and discuss problems, methods, and successful formulas." Starr knew that I had initiated a mass-mailing inquiry to college strength coaches nationwide. The time was ripe for strength coaches throughout the country to become unified in their own professional organization separate from the sphere of powerlifters, weightlifters, and bodybuilders.

The association was proposed for people who wanted to learn more about how to improve performance for athletes. Although many early members had come from the bodybuilding, powerlifting, and weightlifting fields, the emphasis of the new organization was to be kept on strength training.

We had a core of strength coaches who shared a vision for a strength coaches' organization, but how to bring such an organization into being was another matter. Uncertain of the framework, recruitment of members, and legal ramifications for an association, I turned to Nebraska athletic trainer, George Sullivan. Sullivan contacted the president of the National Athletic Trainer's Association (NATA), who invited the strength coaches to attend the upcoming NATA conference in Las Vegas to be held in June, 1978. We soon learned, however, that to start a new association we strength coaches would have to pay double dues. We'd have to pay dues to the NATA as well as to the new strength coaches' association. That didn't seem right to us, but it seemed to be the easiest way to get an association started; we weren't in position yet to hold a convention of our own. In a December, 1977, letter to strength coaches, I announced the first strength coaches' convention for June 14, 1978, to be held in conjunction with the NATA conference June 12 through 15.

But before the NATA convention, Dan Riley—then of Penn State and later of the Washington Redskins and Houston Texans—phoned me and urged that our association forge its own distinct course apart from any link with the NATA. After Dan convinced me, I corresponded again by letter to strength coaches and announced the first annual convention to be held on July 29 and 30, 1978, at the Nebraska Continuing Education Center in Lincoln. Although I was credited as the driving force during the association's infancy, I credit Dan Riley with changing the direction of the organization.

On a convention room floor surrounded by equipment company booths, 75 men and 1 woman confirmed their ambition to form an association. Nebraska athletic director Bob Devaney served as the keynote speaker, with Husker All-American tackle Kelvin Clark providing entertainment, singing a song called "I've Been Everywhere, Boys." A party for all the attendees was held at my house the night before the convention. Mike Arthur, Gary Wade, and Bill Allerheiligen shuttled coaches from the airport to the Nebraska Center. Equipment salesmen displayed their wares, and a banquet dinner was held on the available floor space amidst the strength machinery.

Having recognized a national boom in strength training and the increased number of pro and college teams that had hired strength coaches, we agreed that a need existed to promote the profession and to ensure quality representation. The National Strength Coaches Association (NSCA) was thus established, with its basic purpose being to "unify its members and to facilitate a professional exchange of ideas in the area of strength development as it relates to the improvement of athletic performance and fitness."' Little time was wasted in making these goals a reality.

It's an honor for me to be recognized as the founder of the NSCA. The association has been good for Nebraska, too. Strength and conditioning research was not available early in my career, and I found myself

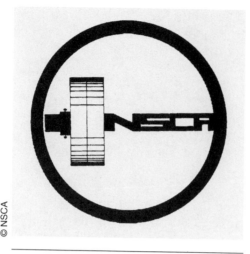

© NSCA

National Strength and Conditioning Association logo.

guessing about the most effective way to train. Nebraska's program is now based on scientific research provided by the NSCA and interpreted by Mike Arthur and Bryan Bailey. Considering the number of schools that pattern their program after Nebraska's, we can't afford to be guessing.

Although I invited 1,000 people from NFL teams, colleges, strength-equipment companies, and the larger high schools from states surrounding Nebraska, only 76 of them attended the first meeting of the NSCA. I was voted the first president and executive director, but after five years I needed more time to focus on my program and facilities at Nebraska. The "national office" was my own desk at Nebraska for the first three years, but eventually it moved off campus, where it was hard for me to keep up with everything.

During the first five years of the NSCA's existence, our membership grew from 76 to 8,500. We changed our name to the National Strength and Conditioning Association to allow for a more diverse membership. After 10 years, membership reached 12,000. By 2004, membership had grown to nearly 29,000. What had begun as a vision had become a reality.

An Important Triumph

When in 1977 the NCAA started to limit the amount of time athletes could train (20 hours a week while in season), many of us feared that position or sport coaches would assume strength-coach duties to gain more time with the athletes. The NCAA also placed a limit on the number of position coaches and assistant sport coaches that schools could have.

In the face of changes being mandated by the NCAA, in 1991 an advocacy committee was formed by the NSCA to bolster the strength-coaching profession. Recognizing early on that the committee was struggling, President Bruno Paluto called and asked me to chair the group for the first three years. As chair, I changed the name of the committee to the College Unity Council and attended several NCAA conventions working toward getting NCAA Propositions 38 and 39 approved to allow athletes unlimited, voluntary training time with strength and conditioning coaches. I targeted the Competitive Safeguards Committee and the Special Committee for Student-Athlete Welfare, Access and Equity. Because of the recognized Certified Strength and Conditioning Specialist (CSCS) certification, the

NSCA Endeavors

Some NSCA endeavors include forming committees to establish scholarships for strength coaches and to bridge the gap between the strength coach and the sport science research laboratory. The NSCA also communicates to members through regional, state, and local workshops. The association sponsors two national conventions annually.

Along with the workshops and conventions, NSCA members communicate with each other via *The NCSA Journal*, a bimonthly publication put out by the association. Early on, I hired Ken Kontor to edit the journal, and he did a tremendous job providing coaches and athletes with information on strength-training methods and procedures. The focus of the journal continues to be on sports conditioning information, dealing with the basic components of conditioning, strength, speed, power, cardiovascular endurance, muscular endurance, flexibility, and agility. Each component receives extensive coverage to provide a well-balanced, total conditioning program specific to individual sports. Weightlifting and powerlifting articles are rarely included.

The NSCA also has its own certification exam, which was introduced in 1985. Dr. Tom Baechle is responsible for developing the knowledge-based exam for strength coaches, which brings credibility to the NSCA. Tom has had a great influence on the strength and conditioning industry. In 1992, his NSCA-certification committee obtained independent board status as a separate corporation. The certification office remains in Lincoln, Nebraska, and moved into a new building in September, 2003.

strength coach was viewed by the NCAA as personnel distinct from the sport or position coach. This triumph in the recognition of the distinct role strength and conditioning coaches play in the preparation of athletes was a big step for strength coaches. The NCAA had rightly recognized that certified strength coaches were needed for the physical health and safety of athletes.

In 1993, Maelu Fleck, Executive Director of the NSCA, announced that another step forward would be a Professional Development Program for curriculums at the collegiate level to distinguish levels of strength and conditioning experience. Unfortunately, this didn't happen, and the CSCS certification program did not recognize persons with experience. As a result, thousands of individuals have the CSCS credential but don't have actual experience coaching. This makes it difficult for administrators hiring strength coaches to determine who is really qualified to be a strength coach.

CSCCa and the Master Strength Coach

In 2001, a group of college strength coaches led by Dr. Chuck Stiggins formed an association to help mentor beginning college strength coaches. The new group, the Collegiate Strength and Conditioning Coaches Association (CSCCa), was formed as a nonprofit, educational, professional organization designed to promote, educate, and service the needs of collegiate strength and conditioning coaches and to help them gain the respect and recognition they deserve. A primary focus is to make sure college strength coaches have the experience they need to do the job (see www.cscca.org for more information about the organization and its services).

I went to the CSCCa's first meeting with the intention of talking them out of starting a new association because I didn't feel another strength coaches' association was necessary. But after just a few minutes of the meeting, it was clear to me the NSCA was not meeting the needs of these college strength coaches. As a result, I became a member of the CSCCa board of directors and outlined for them what developed into the master strength coach mentoring program. Then, along with Mike Arthur, I helped put together a mentoring packet for new coaches.

I now find myself in the awkward position of being a key supporter of the NSCA as well as a board member of the CSCCa. I promised Chuck Stiggins I would not sabotage his association, but my true feeling is that we don't need two associations in this country for strength coaches. We have a specialized profession that demands a professional license and certification. Dr. Baechle has done a tremendous job of giving us the *knowledge* side with the NSCA certification. It's a great start, and Tom deserves a lot of praise for his efforts, but now we need the *practical experience* certification from the master strength coaches of the CSCCa. I would like to see the two associations combined. I would propose that strength coaches start out by gaining certification from Dr. Baechle's CSCS certification commission. This knowledge-based certification is needed for the many individuals interested in strength and conditioning. Then, for those interested in coaching strength and conditioning, I'd like to see Dr. Stiggins' group of master strength coaches become the group to certify all strength coaches (see figure 14.1). Not everyone wants to be a strength coach, but those who do need to gain this additional (experience) certification. In time, I'd expand this certification to include more than just college coaches. High school and professional strength coaches should enjoy the respect that master strength coaches in college are currently enjoying.

As things stand today, the bottom line is that the NSCA is not meeting the mark in producing strength and conditioning professionals with the experience to do the job. The NSCA is an association started *by* strength and conditioning professionals *for* strength and conditioning professionals. It will soon become the largest sports association in the country, and membership will reach nearly 50,000 over the next few years. It has grown

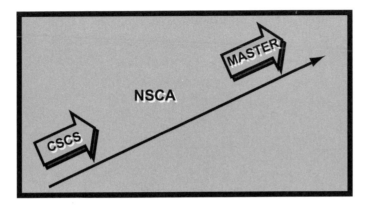

Figure 14.1 Suggested professional certification progression.

so much that it will take a tremendous time commitment to attempt to reorganize and make changes. Getting the NSCA and the CSCCa combined is not likely to happen unless strength coaches demand that it be done. I do hope this occurs and that we can get everything worked out and under one umbrella within the next few years.

Future Landscape in Sports Conditioning

How will athletes be training 5 and 20 years from now? Today we have trainers and therapists who work with injured athletes while strength coaches work with healthy athletes. In the future there will be a new group of strength coaches trained in biomechanics to screen athletes for symmetry and alignment before participation in strength and conditioning programs. The screening will identify athletes who need special exercises to develop proper motor skills. These individuals aren't injured but do have something out of balance that keeps them from being the best athletes they can be. The biomechanical exercises will help prevent injuries caused by muscle imbalance.

Equipment of the Future

Imagine walking up to a power rack to do squats and placing your thumb on a scanning device. The next thing you see is both the height of the bar you're about to lift and the safety level automatically adjusting to the proper height for you. The same scanning device also brings up your program reps and sets for the workout in addition to how much weight you're supposed to use. A sensor on the rack tells the device how much weight is currently on the bar.

You're standing on force plates that graph how much force is being generated from each leg. The speed of the bar is monitored to determine velocity. All of this is videotaped and synchronized with the lifting action so that you can replay the video to see at what point in the lift the most force was generated. During the lift, your posture is monitored to ensure symmetry. To finish off this workout, the certified supervisor places his or her thumb on the scanning device to confirm the sets were done with the correct poundage and with good technique. The device then identifies how many index points and tonnage the workout generated and how these compare to the workout of the previous week and the previous year. A recommendation is then made for the next workout, and all data is stored automatically in the athlete's master file along with his or her posture video and technique video for the day.

Sound exciting? This type of training is just around the corner.

Treadmills of the Future

Bryan Bailey has taken Nebraska into the future by helping develop a unique mobility treadmill capable of running 28 miles an hour uphill or downhill, forward or backward, and featuring an unloading system on which he can dial in how much the athlete should weigh. The unloading system is a huge rectangular frame that stands above the treadmill and has a cable hanging down to support a harness the athlete wears (see figure 14.2). The harness is lifted to take 20 or 30 percent of the bodyweight off their frame. While "unloaded," the athletes can increase their range of motion while taking stress off their spine and joints. These unloading treadmills of the future will not only be computerized but will monitor heart rates and blood pressure. Some already have built-in force plates. They can measure and graph improvement percentages, creating a profile for each athlete.

To improve mobility with the unloading system, Bryan will have an athlete start walking 1.5 to 2 miles an hour and rotate 360 degrees several times as the treadmill continues to run forward or backward. This sideways action improves stability by forcing muscles that aren't accustomed to being prime movers to adjust from the forward action to sideways action without falling down. The overhead cable prevents the athlete from falling more than a few inches.

Rather than having to jog to burn calories, huge athletes can use the unloading system treadmill to train in the correct energy system without stress to their lower back, knees, and ankles. The result is faster running and improved mobility. As athletes have learned to handle more speed with good posture, they have worked up to eight miles per hour while rotating.

It's hard to predict the future landscape of sports conditioning. It's my hope that the NCAA will one day implement rules allowing strength and conditioning professionals to only do drills from the appropriate energy systems for athletes. For example, if a football play lasts only 5 seconds on the average, why would coaches want players to run a mile-and-a-half

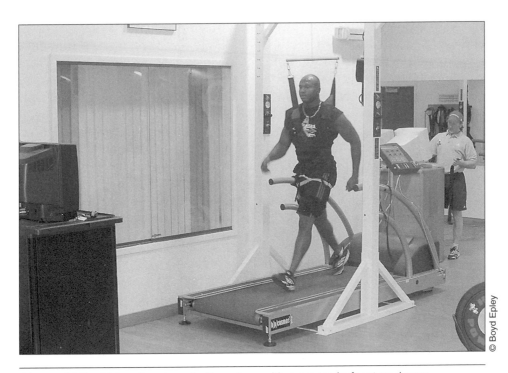

© Boyd Epley

Figure 14.2 Unloading treadmill system with camera in front and rear.

run or mile run or 880-yard run or 440-yard run or 220-yard run or anything that takes them out of the ATP-PC energy system, which has around 6 seconds of fuel in the tank? The tank refills between plays and between drills giving the athlete full power for the next play or drill. If the plays last 5 seconds, the drills should last 5 seconds.

The NCAA safeguards committee has missed the boat on this issue so far. They have focused on ensuring the health of the athlete by requiring medical staff to be present during conditioning sessions. But a better idea would be to require that all drills are done in the correct energy system, which would prevent athletes from being put at risk. Such regulation would force sport coaches and position coaches to learn which drills are appropriate for their athletes and which are not.

The Future of Nutrition

NCAA rules restrict college athletes from banned substances (such as steroids) that increase muscle mass. This means that today's athletes must make the best choices in their training and eating habits to help them fulfill their natural potential. The Nebraska nutrition program, headed by James L. Harris III, RD, is important to the Huskers' success in this area.

Documents indicate a cost of $10 per week to run Nebraska's "Training Table" in 1896. Costs today run over a million dollars per year to operate our "Performance Buffet." James makes a tremendous effort to educate athletes on how to build healthy meals at the Performance Buffet, at home, and when eating out. Team lectures and daily hands-on supervision help educate athletes learn how to build healthy meals. Supervised group shopping trips help athletes make selections that make meal preparation simple, healthy, and economical. Foods at the Performance Buffet are labeled with their nutritional information so that all athletes can make educated decisions when building a meal. James and his Performance nutrition staff plan snacks so that fast foods are not the only convenient option.

After intense bouts of training, many athletes have suppressed appetites. To help these athletes meet their energy needs during training and their recovery needs after training, Nebraska developed the following practices in accordance with NCAA regulations concerning feeding practices and banned substances.

- A sports drink is supplied before or during workouts to minimize decreased work capacity caused by dehydration and fatigue.
- Easily digested sports bars are provided before and during competition to provide a sustained energy source when teams are not prone to consume a sports drink.
- We supply a liquid meal for consumption after training to help ensure adequate substrate and nutrient availability in the blood during the critical phases of recovery immediately after activity.

Nebraska's Future

Strength coaches Dave Kennedy, Mike Arthur, Randy Gobel, Bryan Bailey, Dave Langworthy, Chad Wade, Courtney Carter, Rodger DeGarmo, Clint Dominick, and Mike Greenfield do a tremendous job for the Huskers' athletic programs, and most of them have dedicated their entire strength-training careers to Nebraska. They don't get as much credit for their effort as I would like. Their contribution is seen on the field of play, on the court, and in the pool. Husker fans have become accustomed to seeing Nebraska putting physically dominant teams into competition. Although it's difficult to identify just how much strength contributes in sports, the Performance Team at Nebraska has shown the country that strength can certainly make a difference. As a result, Nebraska has the most recognized strength program in the history of college athletics. I'd like to congratulate our entire Performance Team, past and present, for their tremendous contributions. The "Epley Effect" as described in these pages continues to reach more and more athletes in weight rooms throughout the world. Why? Because of the dedication of the coaches and hard work of the athletes who use the program. Thanks to all of you.

My strength coaching days have come to an end. I've had a great time, and I'd like to take one last opportunity to thank my family for supporting my efforts all these years.

Appendix: Poundage Chart

Husker Power Poundage Chart

1RM	10	10	10	10	8	6	3 (4)	3 (3)	3 (2)	5 (4)	5 (3)	5 (2)
70	45	50	50	35	40	50	55	60	65	50	55	60	65
75	50	50	55	35	45	50	60	65	65	55	60	65	65
80	50	55	60	40	50	55	65	70	70	60	65	70	70
85	55	60	65	40	50	60	70	70	75	65	70	70	75
90	60	65	65	45	55	65	70	75	80	65	70	75	80
95	60	65	70	45	55	65	75	80	85	70	75	80	85
100	65	70	75	50	60	70	80	85	90	75	80	85	90
105	70	75	80	50	65	75	85	90	95	80	85	90	95
110	70	75	80	55	65	75	90	95	100	80	90	95	100
115	75	80	85	55	70	80	90	95	105	85	90	95	105
120	80	85	90	60	70	85	95	100	110	90	95	100	110
125	80	85	95	60	75	85	100	105	110	95	100	105	110
130	85	90	95	65	80	90	105	110	115	95	105	110	115
135	85	95	100	65	80	95	110	115	120	100	110	115	120
140	90	100	105	70	85	100	110	120	125	105	110	120	125
145	95	100	110	70	85	100	115	125	130	110	115	125	130
150	95	105	110	75	90	105	120	125	135	110	120	125	135
155	100	110	115	75	95	110	125	130	140	115	125	130	140
160	105	110	120	80	95	110	130	135	145	120	130	135	145
165	105	115	125	80	100	115	130	140	150	125	130	140	150
170	110	120	125	85	100	120	135	145	155	125	135	145	155
175	115	120	130	85	105	120	140	150	155	130	140	150	155
180	115	125	135	90	110	125	145	155	160	135	145	155	160

(continued)

Husker Power Poundage Chart *(continued)*

							3	3	3	5	5	5
1RM	10	10	10	10	8	6	4	3	2	4	3	2
185	120	130	140	90	110	130	150	155	165	140	150	155	165
190	125	135	140	95	115	135	150	160	170	140	150	160	170
195	125	135	145	95	115	135	155	165	175	145	155	165	175
200	130	140	150	100	120	140	160	170	180	150	160	170	180
205	135	145	155	100	125	145	165	175	185	155	165	175	185
210	135	145	155	105	125	145	170	180	190	155	170	180	190
215	140	150	160	105	130	150	170	180	195	160	170	180	195
220	145	155	165	110	130	155	175	185	200	165	175	185	200
225	145	155	170	110	135	155	180	190	200	170	180	190	200
230	150	160	170	115	140	160	185	195	205	170	185	195	205
235	150	165	175	115	140	165	190	200	210	175	190	200	210
240	155	170	180	120	145	170	190	205	215	180	190	205	215
245	160	170	185	120	145	170	195	210	220	185	195	210	220
250	160	175	185	125	150	175	200	210	225	185	200	210	225
255	165	180	190	125	155	180	205	215	230	190	205	215	230
260	170	180	195	130	155	180	210	220	235	195	210	220	235
265	170	185	200	130	160	185	210	225	240	200	210	225	240
270	175	190	200	135	160	190	215	230	245	200	215	230	245
275	180	190	205	135	165	190	220	235	245	205	220	235	245
280	180	195	210	140	170	195	225	240	250	210	225	240	250
285	185	200	215	140	170	200	230	240	255	215	230	240	255
290	190	205	215	145	175	205	230	245	260	215	230	245	260
295	190	205	220	145	175	205	235	250	265	220	235	250	265
300	195	210	225	150	180	210	240	255	270	225	240	255	270
305	200	215	230	150	185	215	245	260	275	230	245	260	275
310	200	215	230	155	185	215	250	265	280	230	250	265	280
315	205	220	235	155	190	220	250	265	285	235	250	265	285
320	210	225	240	160	190	225	255	270	290	240	255	270	290
325	210	225	245	160	195	225	260	275	290	245	260	275	290
330	215	230	245	165	200	230	265	280	295	245	265	280	295
335	215	235	250	165	200	235	270	285	300	250	270	285	300
340	220	240	255	170	205	240	270	290	305	255	270	290	305
345	225	240	260	170	205	240	275	295	310	260	275	295	310

							3	3	3		5	5	5
1RM	10	10	10	10	8	6	4	3	2		4	3	2
350	225	245	260	175	210	245	280	295	315	260	280	295	315
355	230	250	265	175	215	250	285	300	320	265	285	300	320
360	235	250	270	180	215	250	290	305	325	270	290	305	325
365	235	255	275	180	220	255	290	310	330	275	290	310	330
370	240	260	275	185	220	260	295	315	335	275	295	315	335
375	245	260	280	185	225	260	300	320	335	280	300	320	335
380	245	265	285	190	230	265	305	325	340	285	305	325	340
385	250	270	290	190	230	270	310	325	345	290	310	325	345
390	255	275	290	195	235	275	310	330	350	290	310	330	350
395	255	275	295	195	235	275	315	335	355	295	315	335	355
400	260	280	300	200	240	280	320	340	360	300	320	340	360
405	265	285	305	200	245	285	325	345	365	305	325	345	365
410	265	285	305	205	245	285	330	350	370	305	330	350	370
415	270	290	310	205	250	290	330	350	375	310	330	350	375
420	275	295	315	210	250	295	335	355	380	315	335	355	380
425	275	295	320	210	255	295	340	360	380	320	340	360	380
430	280	300	320	215	260	300	345	365	385	320	345	365	385
435	280	305	325	215	260	305	350	370	390	325	350	370	390
440	285	310	330	220	265	310	350	375	395	330	350	375	395
445	290	310	335	220	265	310	355	380	400	335	355	380	400
450	290	315	335	225	270	315	360	380	405	335	360	380	405
455	295	320	340	225	275	320	365	385	410	340	365	385	410
460	300	320	345	230	275	320	370	390	415	345	370	390	415
465	300	325	350	230	280	325	370	395	420	350	370	395	420
470	305	330	350	235	280	330	375	400	425	350	375	400	425
475	310	330	355	235	285	330	380	405	425	355	380	405	425
480	310	335	360	240	290	335	385	410	430	360	385	410	430
485	315	340	365	240	290	340	390	410	435	365	390	410	435
490	320	345	365	245	295	345	390	415	440	365	390	415	440
495	320	345	370	245	295	345	395	420	445	370	395	420	445
500	325	350	375	250	300	350	400	425	450	375	400	425	450
505	330	355	380	250	305	355	405	430	455	380	405	430	455

(continued)

Husker Power Poundage Chart (continued)

1RM	10	10	10		10	8	6	3 / 4	3 / 3	3 / 2		5 / 4	5 / 3	5 / 2
510	330	355	380		255	305	355	410	435	460		380	410	435	460
515	335	360	385		255	310	360	410	435	465		385	410	435	465
520	340	365	390		260	310	365	415	440	470		390	415	440	470
525	340	365	395		260	315	365	420	445	470		395	420	445	470
530	345	370	395		265	320	370	425	450	475		395	425	450	475
535	345	375	400		265	320	375	430	455	480		400	430	455	480
540	350	380	405		270	325	380	430	460	485		405	430	460	485
545	355	380	410		270	325	380	435	465	490		410	435	465	490
550	355	385	410		275	330	385	440	465	495		410	440	465	495
555	360	390	415		275	335	390	445	470	500		415	445	470	500
560	365	390	420		280	335	390	450	475	505		420	450	475	505
565	365	395	425		280	340	395	450	480	510		425	450	480	510
570	370	400	425		285	340	400	455	485	515		425	455	485	515
575	375	400	430		285	345	400	460	490	515		430	460	490	515
580	375	405	435		290	350	405	465	495	520		435	465	495	520
585	380	410	440		290	350	410	470	495	525		440	470	495	525
590	385	415	440		295	355	415	470	500	530		440	470	500	530
595	385	415	445		295	355	415	475	505	535		445	475	505	535
600	390	420	450		300	360	420	480	510	540		450	480	510	540
605	395	425	455		300	365	425	485	515	545		455	485	515	545
610	395	425	455		305	365	425	490	520	550		455	490	520	550
615	400	430	460		305	370	430	490	520	555		460	490	520	555
620	405	435	465		310	370	435	495	525	560		465	495	525	560
625	405	435	470		310	375	435	500	530	560		470	500	530	560
630	410	440	470		315	380	440	505	535	565		470	505	535	565
635	410	445	475		315	380	445	510	540	570		475	510	540	570
640	415	450	480		320	385	450	510	545	575		480	510	545	575
645	420	450	485		320	385	450	515	550	580		485	515	550	580
650	420	455	485		325	390	455	520	550	585		485	520	550	585
655	425	460	490		325	395	460	525	555	590		490	525	555	590
660	430	460	495		330	395	460	530	560	595		495	530	560	595
665	430	465	500		330	400	465	530	565	600		500	530	565	600
670	435	470	500		335	400	470	535	570	605		500	535	570	605

							3	3	3		5	5	5
1RM	10	10	10	10	8	6	4	3	2		4	3	2
675	440	470	505	335	405	470	540	575	605		505	540	575	605
680	440	475	510	340	410	475	545	580	610		510	545	580	610
685	445	480	515	340	410	480	550	580	615		515	550	580	615
690	450	485	515	345	415	485	550	585	620		515	550	585	620
695	450	485	520	345	415	485	555	590	625		520	555	590	625
700	455	490	525	350	420	490	560	595	630		525	560	595	630
705	460	495	530	350	425	495	565	600	635		530	565	600	635
710	460	495	530	355	425	495	570	605	640		530	570	605	640
715	465	500	535	355	430	500	570	605	645		535	570	605	645
720	470	505	540	360	430	505	575	610	650		540	575	610	650
725	470	505	545	360	435	505	580	615	650		545	580	615	650
730	475	510	545	365	440	510	585	620	655		545	585	620	655
735	475	515	550	365	440	515	590	625	660		550	590	625	660
740	480	520	555	370	445	520	590	630	665		555	590	630	665
745	485	520	560	370	445	520	595	635	670		560	595	635	670
750	485	525	560	375	450	525	600	635	675		560	600	635	675
755	490	530	565	375	455	530	605	640	680		565	605	640	680
760	495	530	570	380	455	530	610	645	685		570	610	645	685
765	495	535	575	380	460	535	610	650	690		575	610	650	690
770	500	540	575	385	460	540	615	655	695		575	615	655	695
775	505	540	580	385	465	540	620	660	695		580	620	660	695
780	505	545	585	390	470	545	625	665	700		585	625	665	700
785	510	550	590	390	470	550	630	665	705		590	630	665	705
790	515	555	590	395	475	555	630	670	710		590	630	670	710
795	515	555	595	395	475	555	635	675	715		595	635	675	715
800	520	560	600	400	480	560	640	680	720		600	640	680	720
805	525	565	605	400	485	565	645	685	725		605	645	685	725
810	525	565	605	405	485	565	650	690	730		605	650	690	730
815	530	570	610	405	490	570	650	690	735		610	650	690	735
820	535	575	615	410	490	575	655	695	740		615	655	695	740
825	535	575	620	410	495	575	660	700	740		620	660	700	740
830	540	580	620	415	500	580	665	705	745		620	665	705	745

(continued)

Husker Power Poundage Chart (continued)

1RM	10	10	10		10	8	6	3 4	3 3	3 2		5 4	5 3	5 2
835	540	585	625		415	500	585	670	710	750		625	670	710	750
840	545	590	630		420	505	590	670	715	755		630	670	715	755
845	550	590	635		420	505	590	675	720	760		635	675	720	760
850	550	595	635		425	510	595	680	720	765		635	680	720	765
855	555	600	640		425	515	600	685	725	770		640	685	725	770
860	560	600	645		430	515	600	690	730	775		645	690	730	775
865	560	605	650		430	520	605	690	735	780		650	690	735	780
870	565	610	650		435	520	610	695	740	785		650	695	740	785
875	570	610	655		435	525	610	700	745	785		655	700	745	785
880	570	615	660		440	530	615	705	750	790		660	705	750	790
885	575	620	665		440	530	620	710	750	795		665	710	750	795
890	580	625	665		445	535	625	710	755	800		665	710	755	800
895	580	625	670		445	535	625	715	760	805		670	715	760	805
900	585	630	675		450	540	630	720	765	810		675	720	765	810
905	590	635	680		450	545	635	725	770	815		680	725	770	815
910	590	635	680		455	545	635	730	775	820		680	730	775	820
915	595	640	685		455	550	640	730	775	825		685	730	775	825
920	600	645	690		460	550	645	735	780	830		690	735	780	830
925	600	645	695		460	555	645	740	785	830		695	740	785	830
930	605	650	695		465	560	650	745	790	835		695	745	790	835
935	605	655	700		465	560	655	750	795	840		700	750	795	840

References

Anderson, J. 1996. *Omaha World Herald,* 7 April.

Callahan, B. 2004. *Lincoln Journal Star,* 25 January.

Hedges, B. 2002. *Lincoln Journal Star,* 23 June, sec. E, p. 3.

Kraemer, W. 2002. "Progression Models in Resistance Training: From the Beginner to the Elite Athlete," NSCA speech, 12 July. Riviera Hotel, Las Vegas, Nevada.

Layden, T. 1998. Power play, *Sports Illustrated*, July.

Mathews, D.K. and E.L. Fox. 1971. *The Physiological Basis of Physical Education and Athletes.* Philadelphia: W.B. Saunders.

Norris, C. M. 2000. *Back Stability*. Champaign, IL: Human Kinetics.

Starr, B. 1978. *The Strongest Shall Survive.* Washington: Fitness Products Limited.

Stone, M., and H. O'Bryant. 1987. *Weight Training: A Scientific Approach.* Minneapolis: Burgess.

Index

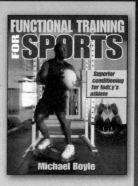
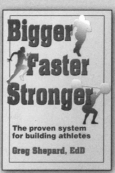
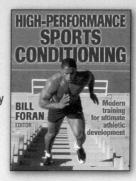

About
the Author

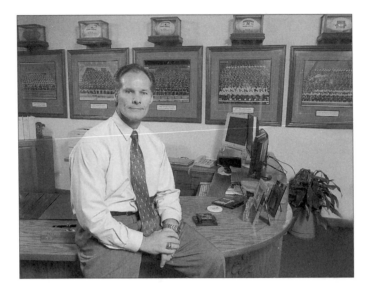

Boyd Epley is the associate athletic director for athletic performance and facility development at the University of Nebraska. A legend at Nebraska and a pioneer in his field, Epley started Husker Power for the Husker football team in 1969. His strength programs have had positive effects on millions of athletes while he has worked behind the scenes with a mission to move athletes to a new level, never be satisfied, always stay focused, and always look for new innovation and research.

In 1969, Epley became the first person to carry the title of strength coach in what was then the Big Eight Conference. In 1978, Epley founded the National Strength and Conditioning Association. He hosted the first national convention and served as president and chairman of the board of directors for five years. In 1980, Epley was the first to be named the national strength coach of the year, and in 1993 he was presented the NSCA's first Lifetime Achievement Award. He was also honored by the Nebraska Football Hall of Fame in 1993 with the Lyell Bremser Award, and in 1999 he was named as one of the top 100 people to have influenced college football in the last 100 years. In 2003 he was named to the College Strength Coaches Hall of Fame.

Epley lives in Lincoln, Nebraska, with his wife, Jane. They have two children, Jay and Jenna.